DEADLY HAZARDS OF FLUORIDATED WATER

In 2018, almost three-quarters of the U.S. population with access to water from public water systems have fluoride, a deadly hazardous waste, in their water. Millions of gallons of this deadly poison are doing irreparable damage by mass medicating everyone who drinks fluoridated water. Let's get this toxic chemical out of America's water supply! If the water in your area is fluoridated, join or start action groups to remove this dangerous chemical now – to save yourself, your family and the lives of future generations!

Here are just a few of the serious health problems caused or worsened by fluoridated water:

- ⬦ **Cancer** in all its deadly forms.
- ⬦ **Digestive system disorders:** Ulcers, colitis, nausea, cirrhosis, constipation, hepatitis and an inability to utilize vitamins B and C.
- ⬦ **Kidney, bladder and urinary disorders.**
- ⬦ **Respiratory and lung disorders:** Tuberculosis, asthma, rhinitis, sinusitis and bronchitis.
- ⬦ **Circulatory diseases:** Arteriosclerosis, heart failure, varicose veins, coronary thrombosis, hypotension and hypertension.
- ⬦ **Blood conditions:** Leukemia, hemophilia and anemia.
- ⬦ **Mental and neurological impairments and disorders:** Alzheimer's, neuroses, psychoses, A.D.D. and multiple sclerosis.
- ⬦ **Eye diseases:** Cataracts, vision proble[...] detached retinae.
- ⬦ **Endocrine dysfunctions:** Diabetes, [...] function of the adrenal, thyroid an[...]
- ⬦ **Skin, nail and hair conditions:** Acne, boils, dermatitis, eczema, alopecia and lupus.
- ⬦ **Bone and joint conditions:** Osteoporosis, bone cancer, arthritis, swollen and aching joints.
- ⬦ **Teeth and gum diseases:** Mottled and darkened teeth, calcium and bone loss.
- ⬦ **Premature and still births, hearing loss and headaches.**

THIS BOOK CAN SAVE YOUR LIFE!

The kind of water you drink can make or break you – your body is 75% water!

More Shocking Facts on Deadly Fluoridated Water

- Fluoridation is mass drug medication.
- Fluorides are toxic to humans, pets and wild animals.
- Fluorides are deadly poisons – in the same class as arsenic.
- Fluorides endanger people who drink a lot of water.
- 1 ppm of fluoride added to water causes urinary output to increase 3ppm in 24 hrs, overburdening the kidneys.
- Fluorides impair the proper metabolism of fats, carbohydrates, proteins and all food eaten.
- Fluorides are cumulative poisons and some serious side effects may not become evident for 20 years or more.
- Fluorides also affects the genes of 2nd and 3rd generations.
- Fluorides depress the immune system, opening the body to disease and health problems.
- Fluoride passes through the placenta and can harm the baby.
- Fluorides interfere with the metabolism of calcium.
- Fluorides can stunt the growth of all living things.
- The U.S. Government strictly regulates the shipping of products containing sodium fluoride.
- Fluorides are concentrated in processed, canned, bottled and dried foods and can cause grave health problems.
- Not enough is known about how fluoride metabolizes.
- Fluorides in the water can ruin photographic films.
- Fluoridation interferes with all living, growing things.
- Measuring the concentration of fluoride in water is very difficult and often inaccurate.
- The equipment used to fluoridate water is expensive while its repair and replacement is a constant, costly problem.

Important, Vital Water Facts To Know:

- Water is more important than food or vitamin supplements. You can go days without them, but you can't survive long without water!
- 30% of Americans drink water that violates federal health standards!
- More than 90% of water companies don't use available technology to remove chemical contaminants and toxins from drinking water!

(B)

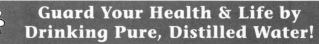
Guard Your Health & Life by Drinking Pure, Distilled Water!

Praises for The Bragg Water Book & The Bragg Healthy Lifestyle

These are just a few of the thousands of testimonials we receive yearly, with folks praising The Bragg Healthy Lifestyle for the rejuvenation benefits they reap – physically, mentally and spiritually.

This revealing Bragg Water book is a real fluoride shocker and should be required knowledge in all medical and dental schools, health related fields, schools, colleges and read worldwide by everyone! Fluoride must be stopped!
– Chris Linville, M.D., New Brunswick, NJ

Health Pioneer Dr. Paul Bragg's work on water and fasting is one of the great contributions to the Healing Wisdom and the Natural Health Movement in the world today.
– Gabriel Cousens, M.D., author,
Conscious Eating & Spiritual Nutrition

Thank you Patricia for our first meeting in London in 1968, when you gave me your fasting book – it got me exercising, walking and eating and drinking more wisely and natural. You were a blessing God-sent! – Reverend Billy Graham

---

A fast with distilled water can help you heal with greater speed; cleanse your liver, kidneys and colon; purify your blood; help you lose excess weight and bloating; flush out toxins; clear the eyes, tongue, and cleanse the breath. Thanks to the Bragg Books for my conversion to the healthy way.
– James Balch, M.D., co-author,
Prescription for Nutritional Healing

In Medical School I read Dr. Bragg's Health Books and they changed my thinking and the path of my life. I founded the Omega Institute. – Steven Rechtschaffen, M.D.
• *www.eomega.com*

"Bragg's Water Book shows the deadly dangers of fluoride to our health. Fluoride is shocking and should be banned!"
– Miles Robinson, M.D.,
Pioneer Food Scientist & Researcher – Santa Barbara, CA

Praises for the Bragg Health Books

Paul Bragg saved my life at age 15 when I attended the Bragg Health Crusade in Oakland. I thank Bragg Healthy Lifestyle for my long, happy, active life sharing health with everyone!
– Jack LaLanne, Bragg Follower to 96½ years

I am truly thrilled by what I've read, and am excited, enthused and confident of my now newer ways to health.
– Ken Cooper, D.C., Narrabi, NSW, Australia

I am eternally grateful for your book. It's made a great difference in my life. I'm sharing it with my friends.
– Carolyn Orfel, Washington, D.C.

"I have been on distilled water for about five months, ever since I read your book. I had pains in my knuckles and a calcium deposit on my left shoulder. These have all left me now; also my bowel elimination is a lot better." – C.A. McFeaters, Pennsylvania

---

"I belong to a Health Club in Buffalo, NY and our members all agree that your shocking informative book on water is the best book on the market. Thank you!" – H.W. Hoffman, New York

---

In San Francisco years ago, Paul Bragg and daughter Patricia were my early inspiration to my health education and career in Health Sciences.
– Jeffery Bland, Ph.D., Famous Health and Food Scientist

I am a champion weight lifter at Muscle Beach for over 55 years and we are all Paul Bragg health and fitness fans.
– Chris Baioa, Santa Monica, California

"For the past few years I have been doing research work on hardening of the arteries and the related problems of ageing. Your great book, *Water – The Shocking Truth*, is far the best and most information I've read on water." – Betty Watts, California

---

Scientists around the world agree the health of the world's precious waters will be one of the most important environmental issues of this century for our planet!
"Clean water for the 21st century and beyond." (page 169)
– Famous Whale Artist Wyland's Ocean Challenge • *wyland.com*

Praises for the Bragg Health Books

When I was a young gymnastics coach at Stanford University, Paul Bragg's words and example inspired me to live a healthy lifestyle. I was 23 then; now I'm over 60, and my own health and fitness serves as a living testimonial to Bragg's wisdom, now carried on by Patricia, his dedicated health crusading daughter.
– Dan Millman, Author, *Way of the Peaceful Warrior*
• *www.peacefulwarrior.com*

I've known the wonderful Bragg Health Books for over 30 years. They are a blessing to me and my family and to all who read them to help make this a healthier world.
– Pastor Mike MacIntosh, Horizon Christian Fellowship

Thank you Paul and Patricia Bragg for my simple, easy to follow Bragg Healthy Lifestyle. You make my days healthy!
– Clint Eastwood, Academy Award Winning Film Producer, Director, Actor and Bragg follower for over 55 years

---

Distilled water is the greatest solvent on earth, the only one that can be taken into the body without damage to the tissues. Distilled water plays the most important part of one's health program in keeping you healthy!
– Dr. Allen Banik, Bragg Admirer and author of *Your Water and Your Health* and *The Choice is Clear*

In contemplating the nature of water I feel that it is the mother, the life of all material manifestation. It is the most flexible and yet the most solid, the most destructive but, next to air, the most necessary. No matter how much it is mixed with other substances, when we distill it, it is cleansed and purified into clean distilled water so that we can drink it to our benefit. – Jeanne Keller, author, *Healing with Water*

There is only one water that is clean and that is steam distilled water! No other substance on our planet does so much to keep us healthy and get us well as this water does.
– James Balch, M.D., author, *Dietary Wellness*

"Your book on water is a masterpiece – A life extender!"
– H. Rosenthal, Ontario, Canada

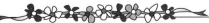

A laugh is just like sunshine, it freshens all the day. – Heart Warmers

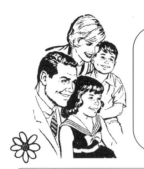

Life's Greatest Treasures
Radiant Health
Physically, Mentally,
Spiritually and Emotionally

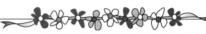

Health, Security and Happiness for You

Can you think of any greater comfort than the confidence that you will not be the victim of fluorides, inorganic minerals, and harmful toxic poisons? This book explains why to keep these destroyers out of your body.

Would it not be a wonderful comfort to you to have this great anxiety removed from your life? How glorious to feel the positive conviction that you can live a long, vibrant, active, healthy fulfilled life! Think of how blessed you'll be once you can teach your children, your relatives and your friends how to live a healthy lifestyle, secure against preventable human miseries and an untimely, early demise! Radiant health is easily attainable by anyone willing to apply these healthy lifestyle principles given in this book.

Bragg Healthy Lifestyle Plan

- *Read, plan, plot, and follow through for supreme health and longevity.*
- *Underline, highlight or dog-ear pages as you read important passages.*
- *Organizing your lifestyle helps you identify what's important in your life.*
- *Be faithful to your health goals everyday for a healthy, strong, happy life.*
- *Write us about your successes following The Bragg Healthy Lifestyle.*
- *Where space allows we have included "words of wisdom" from great minds to motivate and inspire you. Please share some of your favorites with us.*

Patricia Bragg and *Paul C. Bragg*

Dear friend, I wish above all things that thou may prosper and be in health even as the soul prospers. – 3 John 2

Bragg Books are written to inspire and guide you to radiant health and longevity. Remember, the book you don't read won't help. Please often reread our Books and live The Bragg Healthy Lifestyle for a long, happy life!

Patricia Bragg Books

WATER

The Shocking Truth

The Water You're Drinking May Look Safe, But Is It?

PAUL C. BRAGG, N.D., Ph.D.
LIFE EXTENSION SPECIALIST
and
PATRICIA BRAGG
HEALTH CRUSADER & LIFESTYLE EDUCATOR

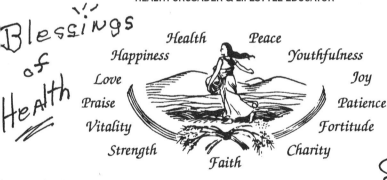

Blessings
of
Health

Health   Peace
Happiness   Youthfulness
Love   Joy
Praise   Patience
Vitality   Fortitude
Strength   Charity
Faith

Patricia

BECOME
A Health Crusader – for a 100% Healthy World for All!

www.PatriciaBraggBooks.com

WATER

The Shocking Truth

The Water You're Drinking May Look Safe, But Is It?

PAUL C. BRAGG, N.D., Ph.D.
LIFE EXTENSION SPECIALIST
and
PATRICIA BRAGG
HEALTH CRUSADER & LIFESTYLE EDUCATOR

Visit our website:
www.PatriciaBraggBooks.com

Thirty first Edition MMXXI
ISBN: 978-0-87790-090-0

Library of Congress Cataloging-in-Publication Data on file with publisher

Published in the United States
HEALTH SCIENCE
7127 Hollister Avenue, Suite 25A, Box 249, Santa Barbara, CA 93117
Toll-Free: (833) 408-1122

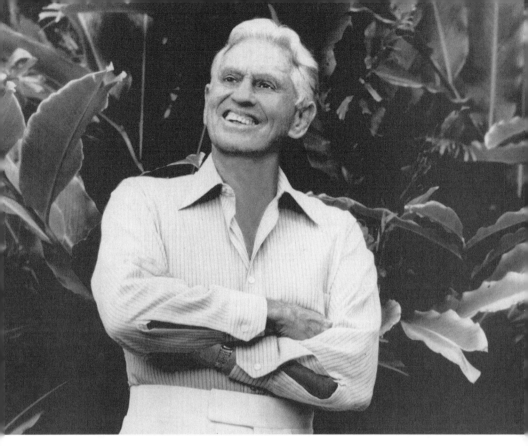

PAUL C. BRAGG, N.D., Ph.D.
World's Leading Healthy Lifestyle Authority

Paul C. Bragg's daughter Patricia and their wonderful, healthy members of the Bragg *Longer Life, Health and Happiness Club* exercised daily on the beautiful Fort DeRussy lawn, at famous Waikiki Beach in Honolulu, Hawaii. On Saturday there were often health lectures on how to live a long, healthy life! The group averaged 50 to 75 per day, depending on the season. From December to March it can go up to 125. Its dedicated leaders carried on the class for over 43 years. Thousands visited the club from around the world and carried the Bragg Health and Fitness Crusade to friends and relatives back home.

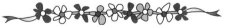

Your body is a non-stop living system, in constant motion 24 hours daily, cleaning, repairing, healing and growing. – Patricia Bragg

To maintain good health, normal weight and increase the good life of radiant health, joy and happiness, the body must be exercised properly (stretching, walking, jogging, biking, swimming, deep breathing, good posture) and nourished with healthy foods. – Paul C. Bragg, N.D., Ph.D.

iii

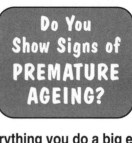

Do You Show Signs of PREMATURE AGEING?

Is everything you do a big effort?

•

Have you started to lose your skin tone?
Your muscle tone? Your energy? Your hair?

•

Do small things irritate you?
Are you forgetful?   Confused?

•

Is your elimination sluggish?

•

Do you have allergies? Joint pains?

•

Do your feet hurt?

•

Do you have aches and pains?

•

Do you get out of breath
when you run or climb stairs?

•

How limber is your back and body?

•

How well do you adjust to cold and heat?

•

Ask yourself these important questions:
Am I healthy and happy?
Do I seem to be slipping and
not quite like myself anymore?
If the answer to these questions are "Yes,"

START TODAY Living The Bragg Healthy Lifestyle!

He who understands nature walks with God. – Edgar Cayce

This Book Was Written to Alert the World to the Importance of Pure Water to Promote Health

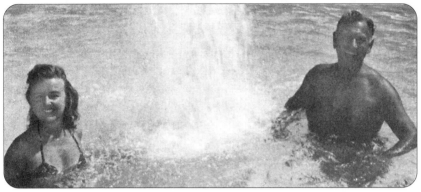

Dr. Paul C. Bragg and his daughter, Patricia, bathing in the bubbling fountain of mineral waters in Desert Hot Springs, California. They believe in mineral spas for swimming and bathing therapy, but strongly advise against fluoride and mineral water for cooking and drinking!

Next to Oxygen, Pure Water is the Most Vital Factor to the Survival of Life!

Humans have survived for as many as 90 days without food, but can live only 72 hours without water before going into a semi-comatose state. Ironically, the kind of water consumed, along with the lack of sufficient water is one of the major substances that brings about arteriosclerosis, illness and premature ageing! Drinking water saturated with inorganic minerals – magnesium carbonate, calcium carbonate and other elements the body cannot use – causes suffering from a variety of unhealthy conditions. Inorganic minerals, toxic chemicals, toxins and contaminants can pollute, clog up and even turn tissues to stone throughout your body, causing pain, illness and even premature death! Distilled water – Mother Nature's flushing agent – helps remove inorganic mineral deposits and toxins from the joints and also helps remove cholesterol and fat from the body. This book unlocks the mysteries of chronic suffering. Over 85 combined years of intense research has gone into this book.

May you be healthy all the days of your life. – Jonathan Swift, 1745

 Bragg Health Books are here to guide you to Super Health!

Cautionary Note and Disclaimer

The information provided here is for educational purposes only. Any decision on your part to read, listen and use this information is your personal choice. The information in this book is not meant to be used to diagnose, prescribe or treat any illness. Please discuss any changes you wish to make to your medical treatment with a qualified, licensed health care provider.

If you are taking medication to control your blood sugar or blood pressure, you may need to reduce the dosage if you significantly restrict your carbohydrate intake. This is best done under the care and supervision of an experienced and qualified licensed health care provider. Anyone who has any other serious illness such as cardiovascular disease, cancer, kidney or liver disease needs to exercise caution if making dietary changes. You should consult your physician for guidance. If you are pregnant or lactating, you should not overly restrict protein or fat intake. Also, young children and teens have much more demanding nutrient needs and should NOT have their protein or fat intake overly restricted.

The information presented in this book is in no way intended as medical advice or a substitute for medical counseling. It is intended only to provide the opinions and ideas of the authors. It is sold with the understanding that the authors are not engaged in rendering medical, health or any other kind of professional services in this book. The reader should consult his or her medical doctor, or any other competent professional, before adopting any of the suggestions in this book, or drawing inferences from it.

The authors disclaim any responsibility for any liability, loss or risk, personal or otherwise, which is incurred as a consequence, directly or indirectly, of the use and application of the contents of this book.

Please consult your physician before beginning this program, and use all of the information the authors suggest in conjunction with the guidance and care of your physician. Your physician should be aware of all medical conditions that you may have, as well as medications and supplements you are taking.

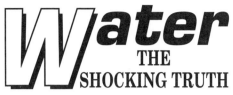
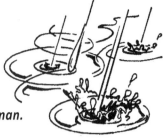

Water
THE
SHOCKING TRUTH

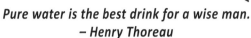

Pure water is the best drink for a wise man.
– Henry Thoreau

Contents

A huge volume of scientific data confirms the protective health role of fruits & vegetables on human health. – Life Extension Magazine (lef.org)

When you sell a man a book you don't just sell him paper, ink and glue, you sell him a whole new life! There's heaven and earth in a real book. The real purpose of books is to trap the mind into its own thinking. – Christopher Morley

Contents

If a man can convince me that I do not think or act right, gladly will I change, for I search after truth. But he is harmed who abideth on still in his ignorance.
– Marcus Aurelius, Roman Emperor

Contents

Contents

The body's need for minerals is largely met through foods, not drinking water. – American Medical Association

Contents

Bragg Books are silent, faithful, health teachers – never tiring, ready night or day to help you help yourself to health!

Relaxation techniques are very important health benefits to the body's general health and cardiovascular system. Such techniques as sitting quietly, deep breathing, meditation and ignoring distracting thoughts can bring down blood pressure and are free of side effects. – Harvard Health Letter

xi

Contents

Water is the Key to All Body Functions!

- Heart
- Circulation
- Digestion
- Bones & Joints

- Muscles
- Metabolism
- Assimilation
- Elimination

- Energy
- Glands
- Sex
- Nerves

Chapter 1

Water – The Shocking Truth!

Pure Water (H2O) is the Essential Fluid Required for Life and Health!

The most important factors that make for a healthier, happier, longer life are:

- Pure, unpolluted air and practicing deep breathing.
- Drinking pure distilled water that is free from harmful chemicals, toxins and inorganic minerals. Ideal is 8 glasses per day for body maintenance and health.
- Eating natural, organically grown foods.

The two most important substances on this earth are air and WATER! Water is perhaps the single most characteristic substance of our miracle planet. It may simultaneously appear in solid, liquid and gaseous forms. It has been adapted as a unit of measure for the specific gravity of all other substances. Water plays important roles in the circulation of the earth's surface elements.

Man must have water or he soon dies! Consider the shipwrecked sailor on a great ocean of salt water – if this man does not get fresh salt-free water, he dies. The man who gets lost in the dry, hot desert soon dies of dehydration if he does not get water. Thirst can drive him insane before he endures an agonizing death.

Certain animals – squirrels, rabbits, etc. that feed on grasses and herbs containing about 85% water never need a drink as long as they can find their natural wild food.

Develop healthy self-esteem to generate positive lifestyle habits that will promote more serenity, peace and love in your life. – Patricia Bragg

The Law of Cause and Effect: An unhealthy lifestyle produces illnesses and disease. Most humans are lacking sufficient water intake to maintain optimum body health! Fact: most people are dehydrated most of their lives! It's vital to have 8 glasses of distilled water daily to operate body functions and achieve The Bragg Healthy Lifestyle for supreme health!
– Paul C. Bragg, N.D., Ph.D.

The World's Water Supply

Location Surface Water	Water cubic miles	% Total Water
Fresh Water Lakes	21,830	007
Saline Lakes	20,490	006
River & Swamp Water	3,261	001
	45,581	.014
Subsurface Water		
Soil moisture & Biological	4,228	0011
Groundwater: Fresh	2,526,000	76
Groundwater: Saline	3,088,000	93
Ground Ice & Permafrost	71,970	022
	5,690,198	1.7131
Ice Caps & Glaciers	5,773,000	1.74
Atmosphere	3,095	001
Oceans	321,000,000	96.54
TOTAL (approx)	**326,776,095**	**100**

Water is distributed in great or small amounts to every part of the earth. All but about 3% of the water is held in oceans; the remainder is found as deep as 3 miles under the earth's crust or as high as 7 miles above the surface, as vapor. The table above shows the quantity and percentage of water in all its habitats.

Mother's milk contains about 87% water; juicy fruits and succulent vegetables also possess almost the same percentage of fluid. Those who consume ample amounts of fresh fruit daily absorb, in addition to about 8 ounces of solid food, at least 3 pints of living, naturally purified water, distilled by Mother Nature.

Water is one of the most important substances on the face of the earth. Without it, all life – from plants to humans and to all animals – would cease to exist!

Water Goes On Forever

Water is absolutely indestructible, but unfortunately easily polluted! Scientists believe that there is not a drop more – nor a drop less – than when shallow water first formed the roundness of the earth with its tidal currents. Volcanic eruptions eventually brought solid rock and earth above the water in the form of mountains. Over time, these new eruptions became the continents.

These tides, conversely, slow the rotation of the earth by a fraction of a second every thousand years. The 24-hour day was probably a four-hour day millions of years ago. Originally the earth probably consisted of hot gases. As it cooled, hydrogen and oxygen atoms fused to form a steamy mist. Much later, the steamy mist fell in endless torrential rains, and the coolness of which eventually solidified the floor of the earth.

The Endless Wonders of Water

Water shapes the earth, controls the climate and provides man with food and a prodigious amount of energy. The body is 75% water (see page 10), which is the source of all life! Water performs and supports the internal body functions of humans, animals and maintains plant life!

Water Penetrates Everywhere

The molecular strength of a drop of water is almost beyond comprehension. Penetrating the lacy roots of a big tree, it climbs upward, pulling after it a chain of water drops. The wind will vaporize the water in the topmost leaves of the tree, carrying it back to the sky to help form a rain-bearing cloud. The same drop may be carried as much as 7 miles above the earth, remaining airborne and becoming purified before dropping with billions of other drops as rain . . . perhaps on an orchard of apples. Or the raindrop (distilled water) may be caught by a group of thirsty sailors shipwrecked on a waterless island. It may fall on the parched ground of Arizona and bring to life a seed that needs only a few days of water to grow. An inch of rain that falls over a square mile of topsoil adds over 17 million gallons of water to the earth.

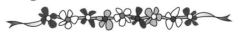

Water is the essential fluid of all life . . . the solvent of our ills or can be the deliverer of a radiant, healthy, long life.

To preserve health is a moral and religious duty, for health is the basis for all social virtues. We can't be as useful when not well.
– Dr. Samuel Johnson, Father of Dictionaries, 1709-1784

The Hydrologic Cycle

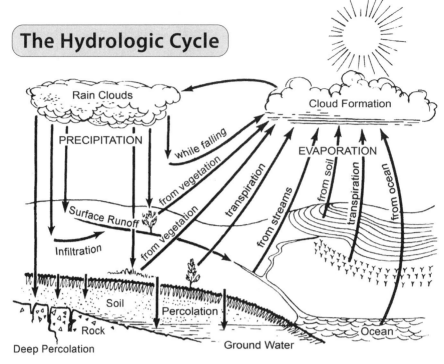

One such raindrop, if it lingers on the surface of the earth, may be re-vaporized and head for the sky in less than a minute. If it penetrates deeply into the ground and enters the water table far below the Sahara Desert, where 150,000 cubic miles of water lies waiting, it may require a century to resurface and become airborne. A solitary drop of water is a strange world indeed.

Hot Mineral Water Under California Desert

Just a few hundred feet below our former desert home in California, there is a raging river of hot mineral water. Wells are sunk down to reach this water, which comes out at a temperature as high as 180°F. This water has been underground for centuries. The water is cooled to a temperature that human beings can tolerate and provides blessed relief to thousands who have aches and pains throughout their bodies. This warm mineral water is very relaxing and therapeutic. People come from all over the world to bathe in its natural, healing warmth!

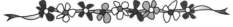

Mother Nature is man's teacher. She unfolds her treasures to his search, unseals his eyes, illuminates his mind and purifies his heart. – Alfred B. Street

We both have had painless bodies, yet still took the time to enjoy these natural hot mineral baths because they are soothing and relaxing to the body and mind and are good preventive medicine.

Angel View Non-profit (formerly Angel View Crippled Children's Hospital) in Desert Hot Springs is world-famous for the help it provides disabled children and adults. It's an inspiration to see their clients swimming in the hot mineral water therapeutic pool! Even though many of the children cannot walk when they arrive, they soon learn how to swim in the pool and this starts to build self-confidence in their little bodies! This hydrotherapy, plus physical therapy, has worked miracles under the pioneering guidance of our good friend, Dr. Frank Edmundson. Our late President and friend, Dwight D. Eisenhower, served on the Board of Directors of this hospital for years.

Oceans and Seas – 97% of Earth's Water

The oceans hold 97% of all the water on earth. They create the enormous tides, waves and winds which crash and slam against the rocky beaches and reduce them to sand. Where volcanic eruptions have flowed to the sea, this volcanic material is reduced to sand over time. That is why the Isles of Hawaii and Tahiti have some beaches of black sand. The sea will always win this battle with the earth! Some Geologists tell us that eventually the mountains may be leveled and swept into the ocean and the cycle of volcanic eruptions will begin again.

Eons ago, the continent-spanning glaciers were so numerous that the level of the seas fell 300 feet and land bridges appeared between England and France. An earthen bridge also emerged between Siberia and Alaska. That may account for some of the mystifying similarities among races, even now widely separated by oceans.

The famed oceanographer, Columbus Iselin, chided science when he wrote, "The sea is producing about as much as the land, yet man is using only about 1% of his food from his salt water environment." Unfortunately, man is more interested in the unknown darkness of our sky and outer space than studying and protecting our vast seas!

Man Cannot Live Without Water

Your existence on earth depends on WATER! Please do not take it for granted! This book gives you an education on the type, amount and value of the perfect water to drink that will work to keep you in good health. Distilled water helps you every day to enjoy a more vital, joyous and prolonged life on our precious earth!

Why the Body Needs Pure Water

The amount of water a body needs depends on the temperature, climate, one's activities and health – the average is 8 glasses. When you drink a glass of water it goes straight to your stomach. Part of the water is absorbed directly into your bloodstream through the walls of your stomach and some of the remainder goes to your intestines to keep the food you eat in a liquid state while it is being absorbed; this water is later absorbed directly into the blood.

Drinking the right kind of water is one of your best natural protections against all kinds of virus infections such as influenza, pneumonia, whooping cough, measles and other infectious diseases. Doctors advise bed-rest and plenty of water for the flu. When the body's tissues and cells are kept well-supplied with ample water, they can fight viral attacks more efficiently. If the body's cells are water-starved, they become shriveled-up, parched and dry, making it easy for viruses and diseases to attack!

Always bear in mind the important functions of the right kind of water in your body. Water is a healthy, vital component of all body fluids, tissues, cells, lymph, blood and glandular secretions. Water holds all nutritive factors in solution and acts as a transportation medium to the various parts of the body for these substances. The mucous membranes need plenty of water to keep them soft and free from friction on their delicate surfaces.

Liquid is necessary for the proper digestion of food! The stomach acts as a powerful churn to break down food into tiny particles! Remember to chew your food thoroughly to help your stomach, for it has no teeth!

6

Water Flushes Toxins Out of the Body

One of the most important functions of water is to flush the toxins and salt from the body. Unfortunately, people the world over now consume large amounts of salt (see pages 108-114). But, from centuries ago to the present day, there are still a few countries that have never known what salt is and whose people are still healthy and happy.

Water is a great flushing agent!

The right kind of water is also Mother Nature's greatest beauty and health tonic! In our long careers as health and fitness advisors to Hollywood's Famous Stars of movies and TV, we have found that when we can persuade the Stars to use the correct liquids they retain a more youthful face and figure longer than people who drink ordinary tap water. Pure distilled water helps keep the body's cells healthier and prevents dehydration. The face and neck remain more free of age lines and wrinkles, and the entire body retains its youthfulness longer!

The Five Big Health Builders
• Air • Water • Sunshine • Food • Exercise

Next to oxygen, water is the most vitally important substance in the body. The adult body is roughly 75% water (see page 10) and excretes water daily through the urine, defecation, perspiration and breathing. The internal temperature of the body is controlled with water.

The average body is 98.6°F. If it rises above this normal temperature one becomes feverish. If it falls below, one is physically under par. Water makes up 83% of the blood in the body and nearly 98% of intestinal, gastric, salivary and pancreatic juices. Most older people become dehydrated and literally dry up due to insufficient water intake. Their skin and hands look parched, withered, dry and old. Look at the wrinkles on their foreheads and around their eyes. A curtain of dry flesh hangs over their eyes. Other unhealthy results and danger signs of dehydration are constipation (see pages 117 and 168), which affects millions, and also burning, irritating urination.

Pure Water is the Greatest Life-Giver!

Pure water is truly one of the greatest gifts to us; a source of life and health. Making sure that we use only water that is safe and uncontaminated (distilled is best) may be one of the greatest health gifts we can give ourselves, our families and friends! Distilled water is the world's best and purest water! It is excellent for detoxification and fasting programs and for cleaning all of our cells, organs and fluids in the body because it helps carry away so many harmful substances!

Water is Important to Superb Health

People who ingest a sufficient amount of the right kinds of liquids (distilled water, fresh organic fruits and vegetables and their juices and ACV Drink, [see recipe page 130]) have better overall health and body functioning, which are most important to Super Health and Long Life.

Whether it be from the natural juices of vegetables, fruits and other foods or from the water of high purity obtained by steam distillation, pure water is essential for health! Your body is constantly working for you . . . breaking down old bone and tissue cells and replacing them with new ones. As the body casts off the old minerals and other waste products of broken-down cells, it must obtain fresh supplies of the essential elements for new cells. Scientists now understand how various kinds of dental problems, different types of arthritis and even some forms of hardening of the arteries (see pages 43 & 137-139) are caused by the various kinds of imbalances in the levels of calcium, phosphorus and magnesium in the body's chemistry.

You have 15 billion powerful brain cells (see pages 84-86) which are 75% water. We strongly believe that the right kind of water in sufficient amounts helps to improve your mind, memory and brain power and makes you think better and more accurately!

Pure distilled water is truly God's greatest gift to us, a source of life and health. – Paul C. Bragg, N.D., Ph. D., Pioneer Health Crusader

We also think that the excessively nervous and/or mentally upset person is so obsessed with his own worries and "hang-ups" that he just forgets to drink sufficient pure water. Instead, he dopes himself with alcohol, tea, coffee, diet cola and soft drinks which only complicate his nervous condition by introducing burning, toxic acid into his stomach with no food or pure water to dilute it. So on top of his nervousness and depression, he suffers from heartburn, sour acid stomach, gas, bloating, enervation and low energy. In place of sufficient pure water, he again dopes up on stimulants, coffee, soft drinks, cigarettes, aspirin, antacids, etc.

Remember that the nerves (see pages 46-48) need the correct amount of water to function properly and smoothly. You can plainly see that it is possible to suffer from water starvation. Here is a simple way that you can help yourself to better health – the Natural Pure Water Way!

The specific reason we wrote this book was to give you the knowledge to select the right kind and amount of water your body so desperately needs! Here is your invitation to enjoy the gift of Super Health, Longevity and Freedom from bodily miseries through following Mother Nature's Eternal Laws combined with the powerful self-health knowledge you are reading.

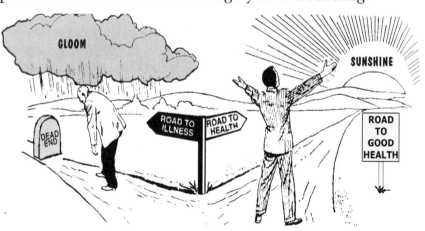

NEGATIVE ⇦ **OR** ⇨ **POSITIVE**

The choice of which road to take is up to you.

You alone decide whether to reach a dead end or live a healthy lifestyle for a long, healthy, happy, active life. – Paul C. Bragg

The 75% Watery Human

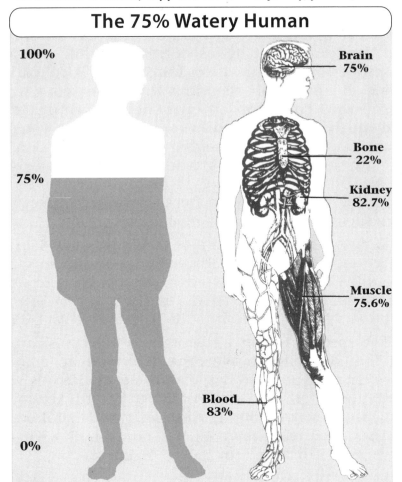

The amount of water in the body, averaging 75%, varies considerably and even from one part of the body to another area (illustration on right). A lean man may hold 75% of his weight in body water, while a woman – because of her larger proportion of water-poor fatty tissues – may be only 52% water. The lowering of water content in the blood is what triggers the hypothalamus, the brain's vital thirst center, to send out its familiar urgent demand for a drink of water! Please obey and drink ample amounts of purified water. By the time you feel thirsty, you're already dehydrated.
– American Running and Fitness Association

Water Percentage in Various Body Parts:

Teeth	10%	Spleen	75.5%
Bones	22%	Lungs	80%
Cartilage	55%	Blood	83%
Red blood corpuscles	68.7%	Bile	86%
Liver	71.5%	Plasma	90%
Brain	75%	Lymph	94%
Muscle tissue	75%	Saliva	95.5%

This chart shows why 8-10 glasses of pure water daily is so important.

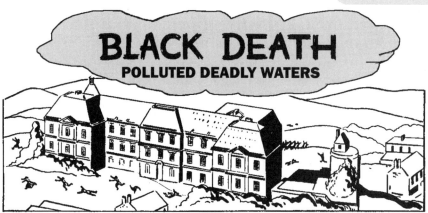

Chapter 2

BLACK DEATH
POLLUTED DEADLY WATERS

The "Black Death" that spread throughout Europe in the 1300s killed one-third of the entire population. This plague was caused by polluted water. Even today in many parts of Europe, the water is unfit to drink. People use bottled water for drinking purposes. Experienced world travelers drink purified bottled water.

"Water! Water! Everywhere – But Not a Safe Drop to Drink!"

Yes, with all the billions of gallons of fresh, sweet water there is on earth, only a fraction of it is fit to drink. A chemical compound known as H2O, water is one of the most abundant and widely distributed substances on the surface of the earth. It occurs naturally in solid, liquid and gaseous states, generally known as ice, snow, water and steam vapor. Water, composed of hydrogen and oxygen, is contained in varying amounts in all natural foods. It's an indispensable solvent needed in all physiological functions in every form of life.

The body requires water that is 100% pure hydrogen and oxygen, free of toxins and inorganic minerals. This water comes from three sources: first, from fresh, organically-grown vegetables and fruits and their juices, which Mother Nature purifies; second, from water distilled and purified by steam; third, from rain water that comes down distilled through unpolluted, clean air.

Shocking Mutations & Death from Polluted Water Must Stop! Deadly chemical pollution is not only mutating but killing millions of animal species worldwide. One USA example: Children in Minnesota discovered and caught frogs displaying horrible mutations, including eyes growing on their knees, four hind legs, etc. Scientists determined that unidentified toxic chemicals in pond and ground water caused these terrible mutations!

Sad fact – much of the world's water today is polluted. It is difficult to find sources of water from rivers, ponds, lakes, streams and even wells and springs that are not polluted or that do not contain traces of toxic industrial chemicals to some degree. Therefore, a great deal of toxic chlorine is added to make this water fit to drink.

But is it really "fit to drink"? Water processing plants use chemical chlorine to destroy bacteria in polluted water. Alum and other inorganic chemicals are also used to cleanse polluted water of dirt and filth. See pages 53-55 and 152-157 for more facts about deadly chlorinated water.

In addition to these inorganic chemicals, a dangerous inorganic substance has been added to drinking water – sodium fluoride. It's the worst chemical ever added knowingly to our drinking water; a terrible crime against public health! Please reread front pages A-B for startling facts about fluoridation (and see pages 21-37).

Inorganic Versus Organic Minerals

Now, let us give you a short lesson in chemistry. There are two kinds of chemicals, inorganic and organic.

The inorganic chemicals like chlorine, alum and sodium fluoride cannot be utilized in a healthy way by the living tissues of the body and can only cause harm!

Our body chemistry is composed of 19 organic minerals, which must come from a living source or one that was once alive. When we eat an apple or any other fruit or vegetable, that substance is composed of living organic minerals. It has a certain length of life after being gathered from the earth, vine or tree. The same goes for animal foods, fish, milk, cheese and eggs.

Everyone has a doctor within himself. We just have to help it in its work. The natural healing force within each one of us is the greatest force in getting well! – Hippocrates, Father of Medicine, 400 B.C.

Health in a human being is the perfection of bodily organization, intellectual energy and moral power. – T.L. Nichols, M.D.

Most Americans' bodies thirst for pure distilled water! Their bodies become sick, prematurely aged, crippled and stiff due to inorganic minerals and chemicalized water and lack of sufficient pure water!

Organic minerals are vitally important in keeping us alive and healthy! If we were cast away on a barren, uninhabited island where nothing was growing, we would slowly starve to death. Even though the soil beneath our feet contains 16 inorganic minerals, our bodies 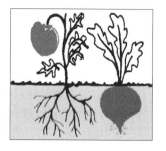 cannot absorb them efficiently enough to sustain life. Only a living plant's roots have the power to extract inorganic minerals from the earth and transform them into useful organic foods to nourish our miracle working bodies.

For years we've heard people say that certain waters were "rich in all the minerals." What kind of minerals are they talking about? Inorganic or organic?

Humans do not have the same chemistry as plants. Only living plants can convert an inorganic mineral into an organic mineral. As you read here, you will learn what harm inorganic minerals can do to your body and brain.

Because of dietary deficiencies, some children and young animals try eating dirt. They can become deathly ill, not from the germs in the dirt, but from the inorganic minerals which can cause sickness and even death!

13

Organically grown fruits and vegetables are grown with all natural methods on organic farms and are far superior nutritionally. The big commercial farms use chemical fertilizers, pesticides and GMO seeds.

Premature old age is a highly toxic condition caused by nutritional and water deficiencies and living an unhealthy lifestyle.

You are a Miracle – Self-Cleansing, Self-Repairing, Self-Healing – Please become aware of "YOU" and be thankful for all your miracle blessings that take place daily! – Paul C. Bragg, N.D., Ph.D.

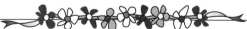

DRINK, DRINK, DRINK. You can easily sweat away more than a quart of water during an hour of strenuous exercise. Sweat rates of nearly a gallon an hour have been reported in some athletes. For optimal hydration during strenuous endurance exercise, drink at least 16-20 ounces of fluid 2 hours before exercising and another 8 ounces 15 to 30 minutes before. While exercising, sip 4-6 ounces every 15 to 20 minutes. Afterwards, drink enough to replace fluid you've sweated off; drink a pint for each pound lost.

Organic Minerals Are Essential to Health

ORGANIC MINERALS. Your minerals must come from an organic source, from something living or that has lived. Humans do not have the same chemistry as plants. Only the living plant has the ability to extract inorganic minerals from the earth and convert them to organic minerals for your body to absorb and utilize.

INORGANIC MINERALS. Inorganic minerals and toxic chemicals in water can create these problems:

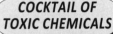

COCKTAIL OF TOXIC CHEMICALS

Chlorine, fluoride, calcium carbonate cadmium, aluminum, trihalomethanes, chloroform, arsenic copper, lead and unpleasant taste

- *Clogs the arteries and small capillaries that are needed to feed and nourish your brain with oxygenated blood; the result is loss of memory and gradual senility and strokes.*

- *Hardens the liver.*

- *Causes kidney stones and gallstones.*

- *Causes arthritis, bone spurs and painful calcified formations in the joints.*

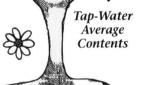

Tap-Water Average Contents

14

Distilled water plays a vital part in the treatment of illness, arthritis, etc. – Dr. Allen E. Banik, author of "Your Water and Your Health" & "The Choice is Clear"

Beware of Dangerous Inorganic Minerals And Toxins in Our Drinking Water

As previously noted, chlorine, alum and other inorganic minerals such as calcium carbonate, magnesium carbonate and potassium carbonate are used to "purify" our drinking water. Keep in mind the human body needs hydrogen and oxygen as natural solvents in its internal chemistry. Therefore our bodies need a constant supply of clean water. Where to get it? Even untreated, so-called "pure" water from springs and wells often contain some traces of inorganic minerals and toxic pollutants from industry, farms, fertilizers, etc.

Most Americans' bodies thirst for pure distilled water! Their bodies become sick, prematurely aged, crippled and stiff due to inorganic minerals and chemicalized water and lack of sufficient pure water! – Paul C. Bragg, N.D., Ph.D., Pioneer World Health Crusader

This is the irony of Mother Nature: that this fluid – without which man can barely exist for more than 72 hours before lapsing into a semi-comatose state, contains in most of its forms the exact inorganic chemicals which bring about the ultimate premature ageing of man and animals. Major aluminum companies want to pollute all our water with sodium fluoride (for more info on fluoride see pages 21-37), their deadly waste product they produce through aluminum processing.

Mankind is Sick and Growing Sicker!

Throughout the whole of recorded history, man has suffered with a variety of miseries, a great many of which can be directly traced to hard, inorganic mineral water. In a Milwaukee museum, we saw the backbones (spines) of Native Americans who lived in the area that is now Wisconsin over a thousand years ago, all with calcification that showed they were victims of arthritis. These Native Americans drank the Lake Michigan water, which is heavily saturated with inorganic calcium carbonate and other inorganic minerals. Their spring and river waters were no better.

15

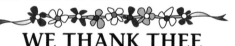

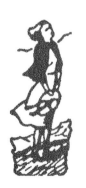

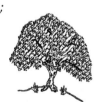

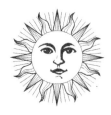

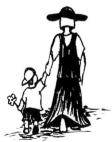

WE THANK THEE

For flowers that bloom about our feet;
For song of bird and hum of bee;
For all things fair we hear or see,
Father in heaven we thank Thee!
For blue of stream and blue of sky;
For pleasant shade of branches high;
For fragrant air and cooling breeze;
For beauty of the blooming trees,
Father in heaven we thank Thee!
For mother love and father care;
For brothers strong and sisters fair;
For love at home and here each day;
For guidance lest we go astray,
Father in heaven we thank Thee!
For this new morning with its light;
For rest and shelter of the night;
For health and food, for love and friends;
For every thing His goodness sends,
Father in heaven we thank Thee!
– Ralph Waldo Emerson

One thing early Native Americans didn't have to worry about, however, was harmful chlorination and fluoridation of their drinking water which would have added more poisons to their already burdened bodies. *Sad fact: by U.S. Law, all Indian Reservations are mandated to have fluoridated water* (page 36). Even mummies of ancient Egypt, some over 2,500 years old, show ravages of arthritis and other diseases due to drinking Nile River water, which is still heavily saturated with inorganic minerals. You can surmise, even ancient people, living under the most natural conditions, suffered and died long before their time! Inorganically mineralized water truly is the universal drink of disease and premature death!

Every time a person turns on the water faucet and drinks water that has been treated and chemicalized with fluoride, chlorine and toxins or is saturated with calcium carbonate and other inorganic minerals, he is jeopardizing his health, his mind, his life and longevity!

U.S. Drinking Water Widely Contaminated

An EPA 3-year study of the nation's drinking water quality found over 200 unregulated chemicals in the tap water of 45 states. U.S. Environmental Working Group analysis of 20 million tap water quality tests found a total of 316 contaminants – including: industrial solvents, weed killers, refrigerants and the rocket fuel component "perchlorate" in water supplied to the public from 2004-2009.

Typical Pollutants Found in Drinking Water:

- **Lead:** which can enter water supplies through corrosive pipes or improper water treatment.
- **Pathogens:** cause disease and are especially crippling to those with weakened immune systems.
- **By-products of chlorine treatment:** such as trihalomethanes and haloacetic acids.
- **Arsenic:** which may cause cancer, serious skin problems, birth defects and reproductive problems.
- **Radon:** a carcinogen linked to lung cancer.

It is also important to remember these pollutants can be absorbed by the body when showering (pages 154-156).

ARSENIC is a semi-metal element in the periodic table. It is odorless and tasteless. It enters drinking water supplies from natural deposits in the earth or from agricultural and industrial practices. Non-cancer effects can include thickening and discoloration of the skin, stomach pain, nausea, vomiting; diarrhea; numbness in hands and feet; partial paralysis; and blindness. Arsenic has been linked to cancer of the bladder, lungs, skin, kidney, nasal passages, liver, and prostate.

The EPA has set the arsenic standard for drinking water at .010 parts per million (10 parts per billion) to protect consumers served by public water systems from the effects of long-term, chronic exposure to arsenic. *Water systems must comply with this standard since Jan. 23, 2006, providing additional protection to millions of Americans.*

LEAD & COPPER enter drinking water primarily through plumbing pipes. Exposure to lead and copper may cause health problems ranging from stomach distress to brain damage. Since June 7, 1991, the EPA publishes a regulation to control lead and copper in drinking water.

The EPA treatment requires systems to monitor drinking water at consumer taps. If lead concentrations exceed an action level of 15 ppb or concentrations of copper exceed an action level of 1.3 ppm in more than 10% of consumer taps sampled, the system must undertake a number of additional actions to control corrosion. The water system agency must inform the public about steps they should take to protect their health and may have to replace lead service water lines under their control.

The EPA provides requirements on what chemicals are found in their drinking water. Water quality reports are necessary "to ensure that Americans have the information they need about the safety of their drinking water." The EPA regulation directs water agencies nationally to provide information such as: •What lakes, underground aquifers or rivers the water comes from. •What contaminants are in the water and whether amounts exceed EPA health standards. •What health risks are posed by contamination when federal standards are exceeded.
– See updates on web: epa.gov/ground-water-and-drinking-water

RADIONUCLIDES are naturally occurring, although the contamination of drinking water sources from human-made nuclear materials can also occur. Most radioactive contaminants are at levels that are low enough to not be considered a public health concern. At higher levels, long-term exposure to radionuclides in drinking water may cause cancer! In addition, exposure to uranium in drinking water may cause toxic effects to the kidneys.

To protect public health, the EPA established drinking water standards for several types of toxic radioactive contaminants combined: radium 226/228 (5 pCi/L); beta emitters (4 millirems); gross alpha standard (15 pCi/L); and uranium (30 ug/L). For more information see web: *epa.gov/ground-water-and-drinking-water*

Where Does Our Drinking Water Come From?

Drinking water can come from different resources. For one, it can be pumped from the ground through wells. This groundwater is then purified, so that it is without contaminants and safe to drink. Drinking water can also be prepared directly from surface water resources, such as rivers, lakes and streams. Usually surface water has to undergo many more purification steps than groundwater to become safe to drink. Preparing drinking water out of surface water is much more expensive due to the additional steps. Still 66% of all people are served by a water system that uses surface water.

Part of our drinking water is pumped from the ground, usually under sand dunes. In sand dunes water can also sink into the ground through the dunes making it naturally purified. This costs much less money than the purification of surface water. Part of our drinking water originates from dune water. See: *www.LennTech.com*

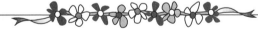

Scientists around the world agree the health of the world's waters will be one of the most important environmental issues of this century!
"Clean water for the 21st century and beyond."
– Wyland, Famous Whale Wall Artist – wyland.com (page 169)

 The power of pure water is the vital chemistry of all life!

The noblest of the elements is water. – Pindar, 476 B.C.

How Is Our Drinking Water Purified?

Treating water to make it suitable to drink is much like wastewater treatment. In areas that depend on surface water it is usually stored in a reservoir for several days, in order to improve clarity and taste by allowing more oxygen from the air to dissolve into it and allowing suspended matter to settle out. The water is then pumped to a purification plant through pipelines, where it is treated, so that it will meet government treatment standards. Usually the water runs through sand filters first and sometimes through activated charcoal, before it is disinfected. Disinfection can be done by bacteria or by adding substances to remove contaminants from the water. The number of purification steps taken depend on the quality of the water that enters the purification plant. In areas with very pure sources of groundwater little treatment is needed. Contact your local water district for more info. See web: *www.LennTech.com*

Dangers In Our Drinking Water

There are several problems that can endanger the quality of our drinking water. A number of these problems are summed up here:

COLIFORM BACTERIA: are a group of micro-organisms that are normally found in the intestinal tract of humans and in warm-blooded animals, and in surface water. When these organisms are detected in drinking water this suggests contamination from a subsurface source such as barnyard run-off. The presence of these bacteria indicate that disease-causing micro-organisms, known as pathogens, may enter the drinking water supply in the same way if one does not take preventive action. Drinking water should be free from coliform.

See web: *doh.wa.gov/portals/1/documents/pubs/331-181.pdf*

It's not uncommon for people to drink tap water laced with 20-30 chemical contaminants. This may be "legal", but is it healthy? – "Scientific American"

There are thousands of case histories of people who have overcome health problems when they began drinking distilled water.
– Dr. Clifford C. Dennison Ed.D., author "Why I Drink Distilled Water"

YEASTS AND VIRUSES: can also endanger the quality of drinking water. They are microbial contaminants that are usually found in surface water. Examples are Giardia and Cryptosporidium. Giardia is a single cell organism that causes gastrointestinal symptoms. Cryptosporidium is a parasite that is considered to be one of the most significant causes of diarrheal disease in humans. In individuals with a normal immune system the disease lasts for several days causing diarrhea, vomiting, stomach cramps and fever. People with weakened immune systems can suffer from far worse symptoms, caused by Cryptosporidium, such as cholera-like illnesses.

NITRATES: in drinking water can cause cyanosis, a reduction of the oxygen carrying capacity of the blood. This is particularly dangerous to infants under six months of age.

LEAD: can enter a water supply from copper pipelines. As the water streams through the pipes, small amounts of lead will dissolve into the water, so that it becomes contaminated. Lead is a toxic substance that can be quickly absorbed in the human body, particularly in those of small children. It can cause lead poisoning.

LEGIONELLA: a bacterium that grows rapidly when water is maintained at a temperature between 86° to 104°F for a longer period of time. This bacterium can be inhaled when water evaporates as it enters the human body through mist, dust, pollution or vapors. The bacteria can cause a flu, known as Pontiac Fever, but also the more deadly illness known as Legionnaires' Disease. See web: *www.cdc.gov/legionella*

BROMATE: a chemical compound that is formed from the reaction between ozone, a disinfectant and bromide. People who drink water containing these by-products develop an increased risk for cancer after several years.

According to a report by the Environmental Working Group (EWG), the top 10 states with the most contaminants in their drinking water were: California, Wisconsin, Arizona, Florida, Washington, Texas, New Jersey, Georgia, Pennsylvania and Ohio. The biggest sources of contaminants were: agriculture, industry and pollution from sprawl and urban runoff.

Men do not die; they kill themselves. – Seneca, Roman Philosopher, 4 B.C.

Chapter 3

The Dangers of Toxic Fluoride

Fluorine is a Deadly Poison

Millions upon millions of innocent people have been brainwashed by the aluminum companies to erroneously believe that adding sodium fluoride to our drinking water will reduce tooth decay in our children. Millions of Americans drink a daily dose of sodium fluoride in their water without knowing of it!

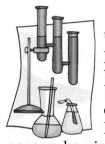 Fluorine, the gangster of the chemical underworld, made the deadly atomic bomb possible. The only scientific way to free the necessary quantities of the fissionable Uranium 235, that is buried in inert mass of its parent U-238, is to force uranium hexafluoride gas through many acres of porous barriers. The next part of the process gradually concentrates the elements, creating deadly "Hex," a destructive vicious hazard from radiation.

Millions of Americans drink water spiked with a sodium fluoride solution: a chemical cousin of fluorine, yet not as toxic as "Hex" . . . but toxic enough, in high concentrations, to be used as a standard roach and rat poison and a deadly insecticide and killing pesticide!

Yet this terrible, deadly sodium fluoride, injected virtually by government edict into drinking water in the proportion of 1.2 parts per million (ppm), has been declared by the United States Public Health Service to be "absolutely safe for all human consumption." Every qualified chemist knows that such "absolute safety" is not only unattainable, but a total illusion!!!

Fluoride is a waste by-product of the fertilizer and aluminum industry and it's also a Part II Poison under the UK Poisons Act 1972.

It's time for the U.S. and the few remaining fluoridating countries, to recognize fluoridation is outdated, and a serious health risk that far outweighs any minor benefits! It violates sound medical ethics and denies freedom of choice! – FluorideAlert.org

The Grim Story Behind Fluoridation

It was in the year 1939 that a famous institute in the eastern part of the United States commissioned their biochemist to find a use for the sodium fluoride wastes produced by aluminum foundries. Some 45 other industries also had fluoride disposal problems. Many were tormented by expensive damage suits arising from the noxious effects of the poison on farmer's livestock and crops! Oil refineries, metal smelters, tile, brick, steel, fertilizer and ceramic plants and the Atomic Energy Commission Installations were all involved! The cost to eliminate this chemical was very exorbitant. Was there no way this by-product could be put to a profitable use?

Now this biochemist was a clever and cunning man. He came up with a big money-making idea: why not dissolve the stuff in drinking water? He had absolutely no medical background and had not conducted any clinical research into the effects of sodium fluoride on our body's chemistry. His idea went over big with companies who were burdened by what to do with sodium fluoride wastes.

The next step was not difficult . . . turn the idea over to clever advertising-marketing companies and let them brainwash the public into believing the greatest health measure in modern times had been discovered. Give a "tall tale" to the gullible American public and if it sounds scientific, they will bite – hook, line and sinker! So they used the tall tale that sodium fluoride in drinking water would prevent tooth decay in children, as they found a Texas town that had naturally occurring fluoride and it seemed fewer dental cavities. The public was eager to hear more. At last, a way to prevent tooth decay! Sadly, most became convinced at first – despite that every smart thinking person knows that tooth decay comes from poor nutrition and especially from the high consumption of all the refined sugar drinks, candy and sugar products!

22

Fluoride is more toxic than lead. Levels of fluoride in water are 67 times higher than permissible lead levels. – Health Action Network Society

---

Researcher Mark Diesendorf assessed 24 studies from 8 countries and found cavity rates had declined equally in fluoridated and non-fluoridated areas, showing that fluoridation isn't necessary! – British Journal "Nature" 1986

Big business and the large professional organizations have a way of sticking together. Remember, they have the power of the media behind them because of the economic control exerted by the publishers' chief source of income – advertising! With the aid of television, radio, newspapers and magazines, the major business, professional and social organizations promoted the 'great merits' of sodium fluoride – although totally false and dangerous – to the innocent, believing American people!

Any person who publicly questioned this poisoning of drinking water with sodium fluoride was called ignorant, uninformed and backward! Most doctors and dentists surrendered to these powerful forces for fear of being discredited by their professional associations! However, you can always find honest and sincere professionals who fight for truth – no matter how others might ridicule them! Extreme pressures were put on all city and state governments to fluoridate drinking water and still are! Big business and large professional organizations, which can act like the Mafia, do not take "No" for an answer! They know how to pressure state, city and water officials to think and take action their way, which is often not for good!

Shocking Historical Fluoride Facts

- Adolf Hitler sought a means to make people docile and suggestible. He discovered that odorless sodium fluoride slowly poisons and makes dormant the small tissue in the brain's left rear occipital lobe that normally helps a person resist domination. Fluoride allows muscles to move one way, but not relax. In large doses fluoride can cause paralysis and death.

- Sodium fluoride is classified with arsenic and cyanide as a dangerous poison and is used in rat poison. Hydrogen fluoride is an industrial pollutant. It is illegal to sell or give away a fluoride pill of 1 mg. Fluoride slowly destroys the body's self-repair and rejuvenation capabilities causing premature ageing, bone damage and deformities.

- Fluoride increases the risk of hip fractures up to 41%. Fluoridation can cause ugly tooth enamel mottling, poor health, Down Syndrome in infants and could increase the growth of dangerous cancer cells.

Is Fluoridation Really in the Best Interest of Public Health?

"First of all, water fluoridation is very bad medicine." Dr. Paul Connett says, "because once you put it in the water, you can't control the dose. You can't control who gets it. There is no oversight. You're allowing a community to do to everyone what a doctor can do to no one . . . force a patient to take a particular medication."

Prior to 1945 when communal water fluoridation in the US took effect, fluoride was actually a known toxin. A 1936 issue of the *Journal of the American Dental Association* stated that fluoride at the 1 ppm (part per million) concentration is as toxic as arsenic and lead. Years later, the *Journal of the American Medical Association* stated in the Sept. 18, 1943 issue that fluorides are poisons that change the permeability of cell membrane by certain enzymes. Additionally, an editorial published in the *Journal for the American Dental Association* on October 1, 1944 stated, "Drinking water containing as little as 1.2 ppm fluoride will cause developmental disturbances. We cannot run the risk of producing such serious systemic disturbances. The potentialities for harm far outweigh those for good."

24

Secondly, water fluoridation is both unnecessary and completely avoidable! Ending water fluoridation is as easy as turning off a spigot! It's not a matter of having to devise costly equipment to somehow take it out of the water supply. Today even promoters of fluoridation say that the major benefits are topical: fluoride works from the outside of the tooth, not from inside of your body, so why swallow it? Why put it in the drinking water when you could just brush your teeth with fluoridated toothpaste if you choose? Please note that we do NOT believe that you should use fluoride in your toothpaste, but are just emphasizing the point that it might work topically but does not work at all when you swallow it! There are far better options for decreasing tooth decay than using a topical poison.

We must all demand safe, purified water!

"Fluoride in the water is essentially an uncontrolled use of a drug."
– Dentist Michael Fleming

Third, water fluoridation is ineffective. There is practically no difference in tooth decay between fluoridated and non-fluoridated countries and no difference between states that have a high or low percentage of their water fluoridated. Meanwhile fluoride can cause significant harm. We know 32% of American children have been overexposed to fluoride. A telltale sign of dental fluorosis in its mildest form is little white specs on the teeth. When it gets more serious, it affects more of the surface of the teeth and becomes colored, yellow and brown mottling and enamel erosion of the teeth (more on page 29).

Fourthly, fluoride breaks down your bones and damages your thyroid. Approximately 50% of the fluoride that you ingest each day ends up accumulating in your bones over a lifetime. So you are steadily increasing the fluoride levels in your bones over time. More info on skeletal fluorosis on page 30. Also fluoride lowers thyroid function. This is a very real and significant concern, especially today as millions of people suffer with low thyroid function.

– from *Huffpost Healthy Living,* Oct. 2010

25

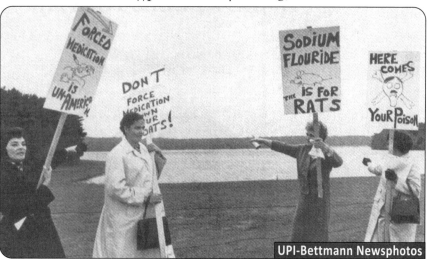

UPI-Bettmann Newsphotos

Who Opposes Water Fluoridation?

#1 Most of the Developed World; #2 Nobel Prize-Winning Scientist; #3 Scientists at the Environmental Protection Agency (EPA); #4 Thousands of Medical and Scientific Professionals; #5 Key Leaders in the Environmental Health Community; #6 Civil Rights Leaders; #7 The Ultimate Consumer Advocate, Ralph Nader; #8 The Majority of Communities in North America; #9 Over 50 Communities Since 2010; #10: Nature – the vast majority of fresh surface water, and the vast majority of plants contain very low levels of fluoride. – *fluoridealert.org*

"The Fluoridation Fiasco" *

In recent years, fluoridation of our water supply has been shown not only ineffective in preventing tooth decay, but it is poisonous to the body! How and why should public health policy and the American media live with and perpetuate this toxic water poisoning sham?

At first, industry could dispose of fluoride legally only in small amounts by selling it to insecticide and rat poison manufacturers. Then a commercial outlet was devised in the mid 1930s when a connection was made between a water supply bearing traces of natural fluoride and lower rates of tooth decay. Even after this connection was proven erroneous, it became a political, not a scientific issue! Many opponents originally started out as proponents, but changed their minds after closer looks at mounting evidence. They started viewing it as a capitalist-style con job of epic proportions poured down American throats.

Some "Fluoridation Fiasco" Facts:

- The Sierra Club found in a study that people in un-fluoridated developing nations have fewer dental caries than those living in industrialized nations. They concluded "fluoride is not essential to dental health."

- In British Columbia, only 11% of the population drinks fluoridated water, as opposed to 40-70% in other Canadian regions. Yet British Columbia has the lowest rate of tooth decay in Canada, with the lowest rates of dental caries occurring in areas of the province where the water is not fluoridated.

- In 1986-87, 39,000 school children between ages 5 and 17, living in 84 areas around the country, were studied. One third of the places were fluoridated, one third were partially fluoridated and one third were not. Results showed no statistically significant differences in dental decay rates between fluoridated and un-fluoridated cities.

- A World Health Organization survey reports a decline of dental decay in Western Europe, which is 98% un-fluoridated. Europe's declining dental decay rates are equal to and sometimes lower than the U.S. rates.

Excerpts from an article by Gary Null called "The Fluoridation Fiasco"

More Shocking "Fluoridation Fiasco" Facts:

- A 1992 University of Arizona study yielded surprising results when they found that "the more fluoride a child drinks, the more cavities appear in the teeth."

- All the Native American Indian Reservations are now fluoridated by law. Children living on them have more dental decay and other oral health problems and diabetes caused by high sugar, refined foods, etc., than do children living in other U.S. communities!

- Most of Western Europe has rejected fluoridation on the grounds that it is unsafe! Sweden's Nobel Medical Institute recommended against fluoridation and the process was banned! The Netherlands outlawed the practice in 1976. France decided against it after consulting with its Pasteur Institute! Germany, rejected the practice because 1 ppm was dangerously "close to the dose at which long-term damage to the human body is to be expected."

- J. William Hirzy, Ph.D., Senior Vice-President of the National Federation of Federal Employees stated in a letter, July 2, 1997 to Jeff Green, of Citizens for Safe Drinking Water, "I am pleased to report that our union, which represents and is comprised of the scientists, lawyers, engineers and other professionals at the headquarters in Washington, D.C. of the US Environmental Protection Agency, has voted to co-sponsor the California Citizen's Petition to prohibit fluoridation. The evidence over the last 11 years indicates a causal link between fluoride and cancer, genetic damage, neurological impairment, bone pathology and lower IQ in children. We conclude that the health and welfare of the public is NOT served by the addition of fluoride to the public water supply!"

Babies exposed to higher levels of fluoride score lower on IQ tests.
– Environmental Health News • childrenshealthdefense.org

FACT: *Fluoride is a dangerous substance and the active ingredient in most insecticides! If ingested, as little as 1/10 of an ounce of fluoride can kill a 100 lb. adult and a 1/100 of an ounce can kill a 10 lb. infant. Studies have shown that exposure to fluoride can cause neurological damage, and an increased risk of bone cancer.* **FICTION:** *Fluoride added to the public water supply strengthens teeth and helps prevent cavities.*

More Shocking "Fluoridation Fiasco" Facts:

- Some fruit juices contain shocking amounts of fluoride, with some brands of grape juice containing much higher levels – up to a highly toxic 6.8 ppm! Also the use of fluoride-containing insecticides in grape crops is a factor in these high levels. Cooking can greatly increase a food's fluoride content. Also, keep in mind that toxic fluoride is also an ingredient in pharmaceuticals, aerosols, insecticides and pesticides. Common fluoride levels in toothpaste are 1000 ppm. When fluoride is ingested, about 93% is absorbed into the bloodstream and what is not excreted is deposited in the bones and teeth of the body – *Shocking Facts!*

- Fluoride use is toxic, absolutely unsafe and should be stopped immediately! The government feels that its central concern is to protect industry, therefore the solution to pollution is dilution! You poison everyone a little bit rather than poison a few people a lot. This way, people don't know what's going on. Any public health official who criticizes the practice of this toxic fluoridation is at risk of losing his job. Shocking: National Toxicology Program Researchers downgraded cancers caused by fluoridation after being coerced by superiors to change their stunning, truthful findings!

- Fluoride has been proven to cause osteosarcoma, a rare bone cancer; squamous-cell carcinoma in the mouth; fluorosis of the teeth; osteosclerosis of the long bones; liver cancer; chromosome aberrations; genetic damage; and skeletal fluorosis and deformities. B. Spittle, author of *Psychopharmacology of Fluoride: A Review* states, "There appears to be strong evidence that chronic exposure to fluoride may be linked with cerebral impairment that affects particularly the concentration and memory in some individuals."

Juice Drinks Contain Dangerous Levels of Fluoride: 42% of commercially prepared juices contain toxic levels of fluoride. Grape juice is especially bad because of the fluoride-containing insecticides used on the grapes.
– Journal of Clinical Pediatric Dentistry

Russian studies back in the 1970s demonstrated that workers suffering from exposure to toxic fluoride in the workplace exhibited signs of impaired mental functioning. – Health Action Network Society – www.hans.org

What is Dental Fluorosis?

Dental Fluorosis: mottling of the tooth enamel, which is permanent once a child's teeth are formed. The staining and mottling happens when fluoride disrupts the process of enamel formation, making it more and more porous. In moderate to severe cases, these porous lesions will extend toward the inner enamel. The porous areas may then flake off, creating visible defects in the enamel. As the fluorosis grows in severity the initial opaque areas turn into yellow or brown discolorations and the teeth may develop pits in the surface. Since the function of your enamel is to protect the dentin and pulp from decay and infection, Dental Fluorosis cannot reasonably be considered a mere cosmetic defect! – *mercola.com*

Proven Fluoride Danger Facts on Teeth!

USE NON-FLUORIDE TOOTHPASTE
Fluoride in toothpaste is absorbed through the lining of the mouth. In only 1-2 brushings, a milligram of fluoride enters your body. – Health Action Network

TOOTH DECAY DECLINE IS UNRELATED TO FLUORIDE
Tooth decay has declined worldwide, with no difference between countries with or without water fluoridation. – Health Action Network

THE SAD, UNNECESSARY EPIDEMIC OF DENTAL FLUOROSIS
This disease, marked by tooth enamel malformation, mottled-discoloration and brittleness, affects 30% of children living in areas with fluoridated water. Only 10% of children in non-fluoridated locations have dental fluorosis.
   – Public Health Service figures

H. DEAN CHANGES HIS MIND – Retracts Fluoridation Endorsement!
H. Trendley Dean, the original promoter of water fluoridation, admitted under oath in 1955 that it doesn't work as a remedy for tooth decay.
   – Fluoride, Vol. 14, No. 3, July 1981

STUDY REVEALS THAT FLUORIDE CAUSES TOOTH DECAY!
Children in India who drank fluoridated water suffered from significantly more tooth decay than children who did not. Especially at risk were children with very little calcium in their diets.
   – "The Journal of the New Zealand Pure Water Association"

CHILDREN POISONED BY TOOTHPASTE
When fluoride toothpaste was first sold in the 1950s, warnings that it should not be used by children under 6 were eliminated from the package – because it damaged sales! When two children in Tacoma, Washington, began to throw up every night before bed, doctors told the parents that their toothpaste was to blame. At last fluoride danger warnings are mandatory on all new fluoride toothpaste labels! – The Fluoride Report

What is Skeletal Fluorosis?

Skeletal Fluorosis: a complicated illness that occurs when too much fluoride has accumulated in your bones. It has a number of stages. The first two stages are pre-clinical, which means you may not feel any symptoms but changes have already taken place in your body.

In the first pre-clinical stage, biochemical changes occur in your blood and bone composition; in the second stage, changes can now be seen in biopsied bone samples. Once you are in the early clinical stage of Skeletal Fluorosis, your symptoms may include:
- Pain in your bones and joints
- Burning, prickling, and tingling in your limbs
- Muscle weakness
- Chronic fatigue
- Gastrointestinal disorders
- Reduced appetite and weight loss

In the second stage of toxic Skeletal Fluorosis you may experience the following unhealthy symptoms:
- Constant pain in your bones and stiff joints
- Anemia
- Brittle bones and Osteosclerosis
- Calcification of tendons, ligaments of ribs or pelvis
- Osteoporosis in the long bones
- Bony spurs may also appear on your limb bones, especially around your knee, elbow, and on the surface of the tibia and ulna

In advanced Skeletal Fluorosis extremities become weak and moving your joints becomes difficult, and vertebrae partially fuse together, effectively crippling you.

Most Skeletal Fluorosis experts agree that ingesting 20 mgs of fluoride a day for 20 years or more can cause crippling Skeletal Fluorosis. Doses as low as 2-5 mgs per day can induce the pre-clinical and earlier clinical stages.

Your risk of Skeletal Fluorosis depends on more than just the level of fluoride in your water. It also depends on your nutritional status, intake of vitamin D and protein, amount of calcium and ratio of calcium to magnesium in your drinking water as well as other factors. – *mercola.com*

Proven Fluoride Danger Facts on Bones!

U.S. HIP FRACTURE RATE HIGHEST IN THE WORLD
The fluoridation of U.S. water is weakening our bones, slowly but surely.
> – U.S. National Research Council and Townsend Letter for Doctors

FLUORIDE AND OSTEOPOROSIS
Seniors living in areas with elevated fluoride levels in drinking water suffer up to 41% more hip fractures. In a study of 3,578 senior citizens, those who lived in areas with fluoridated water had a much greater risk of hip fractures.
> – Journal of the American Medical Association

FLUORIDE AND BONE CANCER
One study concluded that males under the age of 20 who live in areas with fluoridated water were 6 times more likely to suffer from bone cancer than males who don't. – New Jersey Department of Health

FLUORIDATED WATER INCREASES BONE CANCER RISK
In a study conducted by New Jersey Department of Health, young men who drank fluoridated water had a higher incidence of bone cancer. – The Record

OSTEOPOROSIS, CALCIUM AND FLUORIDE
U.S. National Institutes of Health (NIH) gathered an expert panel to discuss causes of the rising epidemic of bone fractures in the elderly. Although the evidence clearly shows that calcium supplements don't help, and also shows that fluoride is terrible for the bones, NIH simply recommended an increase in the recommended daily allowance of calcium. – The Fluoride Report

FLUORIDE ACTUALLY REDUCES BONE STRENGTH, Instead of Increasing It!
In a 5 year U.S. study conducted to test fluoride as a treatment for osteoporosis, bone density was actually decreased 45%, therefore causing osteoporosis, rather than preventing it! The doses used were very close to the amount Americans take in over a 50 year span. – Bone, Vol. 15, May – June 1994

OVERWHELMING EVIDENCE, FLUORIDE WEAKENS BONES:
Dr. John Lee showed that ". . . 7 out of 10 recent studies show a clear correlation between bone fractures and water fluoridation. One study involved 560,000 women over 65." – The Fluoride Report, Sept., 1994

HIGHLY PUBLICIZED FLUORIDE U.S. STUDIES SHOW MEDICAL MISTAKE
The high doses of sodium fluoride used in clinical studies of this drug are known to lead to a condition called osteofluorosis. This means abnormal bone growth and calcification of tendons and ligaments. Although this may help prevent spinal fracture and compression, it also increases risk of hip fracture and causes arthritis-like pain.
> – Open letter from famous pioneer Dr. John R. Lee to Dr. Charles Y.C. Pak, regarding Dr. Pak's study on sodium fluoride in the "Annals of Internal Medicine"

CHECK FOLLOWING WEBSITES FOR FLUORIDE UPDATES:
- *www.FluorideAlert.org* • *www.bruha.com/fluoride*
- *www.fluoridation.com*
- *www.dentalwellness4u.com/oralhealth/fluoride.html*

Studies Show Fluoride Causes Cancer and Many Other Health Problems*

- Studies show that fluoridation is causing an increase in bone cancer and deaths among males under 20.
- The growing increase in osteosarcoma is attributable to an increase in toxic fluoride.
- Evidence shows that fluoridation is causing an increase in oral (mouth) cancer. Don't use fluoride toothpastes or give your dentist consent to do fluoride gel treatments or use fluoride polishing paste!
- Fluoride has been linked to many health problems:
  - bone and oral cancers in humans (even in animals)
  - an ability to inhibit the DNA repair enzyme system
  - accelerates tumor growth and inhibits immune system
  - causes genetic damage in cell lines and induces melanotic tumors and fibrosarcomas.
  - other tumors/cancers strongly indicate fluoride has generalized effect of increasing them overall.
- According to our estimates, thousands of people in the United States die of cancer each year due to fluoridation of their public drinking water.

32

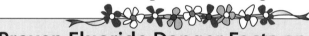

Proven Fluoride Danger Facts on Health!

FLUORIDE AFFECTS IMMUNE FUNCTION
Because of its disabling effects on enzyme activity, fluoride reduces resistance against infection. – Complementary Medical Research

FLUORIDE ADVERSELY AFFECTS CENTRAL NERVOUS SYSTEM
Scientific studies link fluoride to learning disabilities and coordination problems. – Townsend Letter for Doctors & Patients

FLUORIDE AND DECREASING BIRTH RATES
Fluoride is found to decrease fertility in studies of humans and even animals. – Journal of Toxicology and Environmental Health

FLUORIDE CAN SUBTLY ALTER ENDOCRINE (THYROID, ETC.) FUNCTION
Especially in the thyroid – the gland that regulates growth and metabolism. – Scientific American Study

Health risks associated with current fluoride intake (exceeds 6 mg/day) can be described in a nutshell: An intake of 5 mg/day will cause average individuals to develop crippling deformities of the spine and major joints within a lifetime.

*****Excerpt from "Fluoride, The Aging Factor" – by Dr. John Yiamouyiannis*

How Much Fluoride Are You Exposed To?*

In 1962 the US Public Health Service set fluoride levels of 0.7 to 1.2 parts per million (ppm) in drinking water as the ideal range to prevent dental cavities with minimal dental fluorosis. The EPA took over the Public Health Services responsibility for regulating contaminants in drinking water in 1975. In 1986 they relaxed the maximum contamination level to 4 ppm. Some adverse health effects can occur at levels of about 1 ppm and they are more pronounced and wide-spread at levels near 4 ppm.

Although you may not know it, you are exposed to fluoride from many other surprising sources including:

- Foods, drinks, soups, and breads processed with fluoridated water
- Mechanically de-boned meat
- Pesticide residue on foods
- Pharmaceutical drugs
- Bottled baby foods and bottled instant teas

Fluoride Danger in More Than Drinking Water:

- **Pepsi, Coca-Cola and other soda drinks** – *not only because of the water used, but also the fluoride concentrations in the phosphate syrup.*
- **Cereals and other processed foods** – *because of pesticides on the grains, and evaporation of the water used, leaving fluoride concentrations on many products. (Wheaties and Shredded Wheat were analyzed at a high 9.4 times stronger level than the concentration in fluoridated water.)*
- **Fruit Juices** *especially non-organic concentrates from Florida, even ones that are labeled 100% juice because of allowed fluoride based pesticides.*
- **Non-organic produce** *has pesticide residues in scary concentrations. The pesticide Cryolite (sodium aluminum fluoride) which is the favored killer, is allowed on the following produce: iceberg and romaine lettuces, potatoes, cabbage, tomatoes and grapes (raisins).*
- **Nuts and products coming from out of country** *are warehoused in buildings fumigated with sulfuryl fluoride to exterminate termites.*
- **Black and green (caffeine) teas** – *ask for caffeine-free green teas (instant, mixes, etc.) – most tea plants grown on toxic fluoride soils.*
- **Scotchgard** *(toxic fabric stain protector),* **Gore-Tex** *(waterproof fabric), and* **Teflon** *(in cooking pans) are all dangerous fluoride-based toxic products.*
- **Medications** – *such as Prozac, Zoloft, Cipro, Flurazepam, Paxil, Diflucan, Lipitor, Celebrex, Prevacid, Prolixin, Flonase, Paxipam and many more.*
  See web: www.slweb.org/ftrcfluorinatedpharm.html

There are no regulations on fluoride content of processed foods. Many packaged foods are loaded with deadly fluoride. – Health Action Network

*Excerpt from Dr. Mercola – www.mercola.com

Don't Take Drugs with Dangerous Fluoride

Some prescription drugs contain fluoride compounds. These fluorinated drugs have been found to cause serious side effects, such as interfering with thyroid activity and causing liver disease. Chronic hepatitis has also been indicated as a side effect of these drugs.

Fluoridated drugs have a tendency to affect elimination of other drugs, due to their impact on your enzymes. By inhibiting certain enzymes, the chemicals of other drugs can accumulate to dangerous levels in your body, causing a number of potentially deadly scenarios. For a list of drugs with fluoride, web: *slweb.org/ftrcfluorinatedpharm.html*.

Danger – Don't Drink Water Contaminated with Sodium Fluoride

Fluoride is one of the most potent poisons known to man. Selling this poison swells bank accounts of big companies who, in turn, often pay big dividends to their stockholders. This money is made by selling an industrial waste by-product! All these industries had to do, using media and powerful lobbies, was brainwash the U.S. public into accepting their false statements that fluoride added to their water would prevent tooth decay.

Caution: Toxic Water Chemical Drink

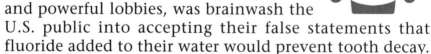

Drinking water in most U.S. cities is being fluoridated due to powerful organizations who are sponsoring this mass poisoning. In our opinion, many early deaths today are caused by premature damage to our arteries, heart, lungs, liver, brain and other vital organs, due to sodium fluoride!

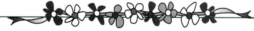

Keep Toxic Fluoride Out of Your Water! *Most water Americans drink has fluoride in it, including tap, bottled and canned drinks and foods! Now, the ADA (American Dental Association) is insisting that the FDA mandate the addition of fluoride to all bottled waters! Defend your right to drink pure, non-fluoridated tap and bottled waters! Challenge and stop local and state water fluoridation policies! Call, write, fax or e-mail all your state officials and congress people and send them a copy of this revealing book.*

The fluoride added to your drinking water is NOT pharmaceutical grade. It is a toxic industrial waste product. – www.mercola.com

URGENT FACTS: Shut Down Fluoridation Now!

SIGNATURES OF HEALTH PROFESSIONALS AGAINST FLUORIDE: *The Fluoride Action Network, as of May 2011, has gathered over 4,500 signatures of health professionals world-wide who are working to end fluoridation of water systems. The signers included doctors, nurses, dentists and scientist. Among the signers is Arvid Carlsson, Nobel Laureate for Physiology of Medicine; the current president and 6 past presidents of the International Academy of Oral Medicine and Toxicology; 3 scientist from the U.S. Environmental Protection Agency (EPA); Dr. Vyvyan Howard, Past President of Swedish Doctors for the Environment; William Marcus, Ph.D. and former chief toxicologist, EPA Water Division; and Lynn Margulis, Ph.D., recipient of the National Medal of Science. – See web: FluorideAlert.org*

HOW THE EPA IS SPENDING YOUR TAX DOLLARS: *When brave Dr. Bill Marcus won back his job with the EPA after being fired for blowing the whistle on the cover-up of fluoride's hazards, the EPA refused to pay interest on his 2 years of lost wages. While the lawyers haggle, the whole sum is being withheld, and guess who's paying for the EPA's lawyers? – The Fluoride Report*

ENVIRONMENTAL PROTECTION AGENCY INFIGHTING: *EPA toxicologists have long been asking that the standards for water fluoridation be revised, while EPA administrators continue to reject their warnings and have even disciplined employees who have honestly spoken out. – The Pittsburgh Press*

35

FLUORIDE HAS NEVER RECEIVED FDA APPROVAL: *and wouldn't pass if it were subjected to the FDA's standards of safety and effectiveness. It's more toxic than lead by the EPA's standards and accumulates in the body. The maximum allowable lead in drinking water is 0.015 mg/liter; the maximum allowable fluoride is 4.000 mg/liter. – Health Action Network Society – www.hans.org*

HEALTH VIOLATION OF MEDICAL ETHICS: *Fluoride is a pharmacologically active substance unrelated to water purification. There is no possibility of obtaining individual informed consent for medication with this experimental drug when it is placed in a public water system. For these reasons, fluoridation violates the "Nuremberg Code of Medical Ethics" and Human Rights.*
     – Health Action Network Society – www.hans.org

FLUORIDATION IS BIG BUSINESS: *Despite the fact that it doesn't actually prevent tooth decay in children or adults, government officials still devote our tax dollars to fluoridation. Several other countries tried it and stopped when their research showed that the risks far outweighed the benefits. In the US, the big companies that make huge profits from selling this toxic waste material are so powerful that the facts are swept under the rug. – "Let's Live!" May 1996.*
(This magazine, originally called "California Health News", was started by Paul C. Bragg, who changed the name because, he said, "Everybody wants to – Let's Live!".

Read and reread this Water book carefully! More than 85 combined years of research has gone into acquiring and compiling this vital information for your health.

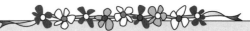

Danger – Toxic Fluoride is Poison!

FLUORIDATION INCREASES LEAD CONTAMINATION: *Fluoride leaches lead from plumbing and water mains. In Tacoma, Washington, where lead content of water had risen above EPA limits, fluoridation was halted because of equipment failure. Officials were surprised at the resulting 50% drop in lead contamination.*
  – Letter from C.R. Myrick, Water Quality Coordinator, Tacoma, WA

MOHAWK INDIANS' FLUORIDE TRAGEDY: *In the period from 1960 to 1975, a Mohawk Indian tribe in the Northeast U.S. was all but obliterated by fluoride contamination. Cows, fish and children all suffered from tooth and bone deformities caused by wastes from two major metals manufacturers. (Now all Native American Indian reservations have fluoridated water!)*
  – "Fluoride: Commie Plot or Capitalist Ploy?" by Joel Griffiths

FLUORIDE IS HIGHLY TOXIC: *Fact is that fluoride is more toxic than lead and just slightly less toxic than the killer arsenic. – Gary Null, "The Fluoridation Fiasco"*

FLUORIDATION ACCIDENTS SWEPT UNDER THE RUG: *Toxic spills of fluoride in drinking water have happened in several communities, but were never publicized. Nausea, vomiting, diarrhea and deaths occurred. – Townsend Letter for Doctors*

FLUORIDE – AN INDUSTRIAL WASTE: *The fluoride in your water is actually toxic waste left over after the manufacture of aluminum and chemical fertilizers.*
  – Dr. John Yiamouyiannis, author of "Fluoride, The Aging Factor"

DID YOU KNOW: *that a family-size tube of fluoridated toothpaste contains enough fluoride to kill a 25-pound child? – www.mercola.com*

Worldwide Fluoridation

Amazingly, the U.S. is only one of 5 countries in the entire developed world that fluoridates more than 64% of their drinking water supply. Canada fluoridates about 40%, in Europe only Ireland (73%), Poland (1%), Serbia (3%), Spain (11%), and the UK (10%). Most developed countries, including Japan and 97% of the Western European population do not consume fluoridated water, and yet, according to World Health Organization data their teeth are just as good, if not better than those of Americans!

In the U.S., sadly, about 71% of public water supplies are fluoridated! This equates to approximately 185 million people, which is over half the number of people drinking artificially fluoridated water worldwide. Some countries have areas with high natural fluoride levels in the water. These include India, China and parts of Africa. In these countries measures are being taken to remove the fluoride because of the health problems that fluoride can cause!

The only known way to remove fluoride from water is by using a reverse osmosis filter or distillation. A simple carbon filter will not remove fluoride.

14 Nobel Prize Winners Oppose Fluoridation

Dr. Arvid Carlsson, Prize in Medicine, Oct. 2000, *for his work on the brain. He played a prominent role in banning fluoridation in Sweden*

Dr. Giulio Natta, Prize in Chemistry, 1963, *Director Industrial Chemistry Research Center Polytechnic Institute of Milan, Italy*

Dr. Joshua Lederberg, Prize in Medicine, 1958, *WHO's Advisory Health Research Council, U.S. National Medal of Science, 1989, Former Chairman of Cancer Panel of National Academy of Science, U.S.*

Sir Cyril Norman Hinshelwood, Prize in Chemistry, 1956, *O.M., M.A., D.Sc., F.R.S., Oxford University, England*

Nikolay Nikolaevich Semenov, Prize in Chemistry, 1956, *D.Sc., Director Institute of Chemical Physics, Moscow, Professor Leningrad Polytechnic Institute, member USSR Academy of Science, member Chemical Society of England & Royal Society of England*

Hugo Theorell, Prize in Medicine, 1955, *M.C., Director, Bio-Chemistry Department, Nobel Medical Institute, President Swedish Medical Association. Stated hazards of fluoridation in a report to the Swedish Royal Medical Board*

Walter Rudolf Hess, Prize in Medicine, 1949, *D.Sc., Professor of Physiology and Director of Physiological Institute, University of Zurich, Switzerland*

37

Sir Robert Robinson, Prize in Chemistry, 1947, *O.M., D.Sc., F.R.I.C., F.R.S., Director Shell Chemical Co., Professor of Chemistry, Oxford University, England*

James B. Sumner, Prize in Chemistry, 1946, *Director of Enzyme Chemistry, Dept. of Biochemistry & Nutrition, Cornell University, U.S.*

Professor Artturi I. Virtanen, Prize in Chemistry, 1945, *Director Biochemical Institute, Helsinki, President Finnish State Academy of Sciences and Art, Finland*

Adolf J. Butenandt, Prize in Chemistry, 1939, *Ph.D., Director Max Planck Institute of Biochemistry, Professor of Physiological Chemistry, Munich University, Germany*

Corneille Jean Francois Heymans, Prize in Medicine, 1938, *M.D., Professor of Pharmacology, Pharmacodynamics and Toxicology, Director Heymans Institute of Pharmacology & Therapeutics, Belgium*

William O. Murphy, Prize in Medicine, 1934, *M.D., D.Sc., Lecturer on Medicine, emeritus Harvard Medical School, consultant in hematology, Peter Bent Brigham Hospital, Boston, U.S.*

Hans von Euler-Chelpin, Prize in Chemistry, 1929, *Stockholm University, President Chemical Society, Director Institute for Research in Organic Chemistry, Stockholm, Sweden*

Mother Nature Loves You To Enjoy Her Beauty

Let me look upward
into the branches
Of the towering oak
And know that it grew
slowly and well.

Give me, amidst
the confusion
of my day
The calmness of the
everlasting hills.

Let me pause
to look at a flower,
to smell a rose —
God's autograph,
to chat with a friend,
to read a few lines
from a good book.

Break the tensions
of my nerves
With the soothing music
of singing streams
and gentle rains
That live in
my memory.

Follow steps of the godly,
and stay on the right path
to enjoy life to the fullest.
— Proverbs 2:20-21

38

Open your eyes to behold wondrous things out of Thy law. – Psalm 119:18

Chapter 4

We Live in a Sick, Sick World
(How Toxic Water Can Make You Sick)

We are independent researchers and health crusaders for the truth. We're loners. No one controls what we say. No organization dictates to us! We have no financial master to serve; therefore we can give you the plain, honest truth. We love inspiring and guiding you with our simple, easy-to-follow Bragg Healthy Lifestyle, so you can enjoy a long, vibrantly youthful life! We've spent our lives researching and studying human health. We've been trying to understand why people become sick, prematurely old, senile and die long before their time!

It's our conclusion that many make themselves sick and shorten their lives by consuming unhealthy toxic water and unhealthy commercial foods! Plus, many use tobacco and also consume powerful stimulants such as alcohol, coffee, diet and sugared colas high in fluoride. They also eat high concentrations of refined white sugar and its products, refined white flour products such as white bread, pasta, white rice and salt and salted foods. They often overeat, mostly refined, devitalized, dead

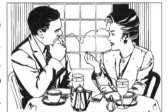

Foods can make or break your health. You can dig your grave with your knife, fork and spoon! Use Caution in what you eat and drink.

foods, dairy, meat and saturated fats! These are the killers that fill the arteries with waxy, clogging cholesterol (read Bragg *Healthy Heart* Book, see page 194).

These bad, unhealthy habits – plus lack of exercise, sunlight, fresh air – adds up to physical unfitness. 97% of people today are physically unfit, 65% are overweight! Most people eat such an unhealthy diet that they suffer from sickness and fatigue. They drag around all day and at night are forced to take sleeping pills to sleep. When awake, they take "pep pills" and coffee to stay awake and keep going!

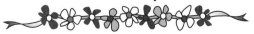

Change your mind – change to a healthy lifestyle and your life and body will sparkle with health and joy! – Patricia Bragg

Physical fatigue and weariness make them more inactive than ever. They just don't have the "Go Power" to lead very active physical lives. As a consequence, their exterior as well as interior muscles suffer from increasing flabbiness. The greatest "disease" today is the physical deterioration of the human body at all ages.

Let's take a good, hard look at our young people. Never in the entire history of the world have so many drugs been used by people under thirty! Why do young people turn to drugs to keep them going? Just take a look at the "junk" and "trash" they eat – that tells the entire sad story! They do not derive enough nutrients, vitamins and minerals from their daily diet! In their ignorance, they try to gain energy by using harmful stimulants such as coffee, sugared drinks, tobacco, alcohol

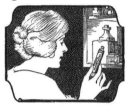

Troubled by Headaches?

We are a nation of pill takers. Every 24 hours between 50-75 tons of pain killers and other tonics are consumed.

40

and drugs. These deficient, "dope addicts" are in danger of having children who are born sickly, some with breathing, asthma and birth defects!

For many people, health is something they value only when they have lost it or are in danger of losing it. We repeat, "We live in a sick, sick, world – and it's getting sicker every day!" Take heed, repent and change now!

"Health" is an old Anglo-Saxon word meaning "soundness." The ancient Greek concept of "a sound mind in a sound body" (*mens sana in corpore sano*) gives the true picture of health. We have to place the adjective "good" with this word "health" only when we contrast it with the phrase "ill health" or "lack of soundness."

The natural healing force within you is the greatest force in getting well.
– Hippocrates, Father of Medicine, 400 B.C.

"Allowing coal polluters to fill our rivers and lakes with this witches brew of toxic chemicals threatens public health and diminishes the quality of life for all Americans." – Robert F. Kennedy, Jr., President of Waterkeeper Alliance • www.WaterKeeper.org

A healthy, energetic body and an alert, keen, healthy mind make it possible for human beings to cope with and bear the frustrations, worries, cares, tensions and stresses of life and yet enjoy life and the joys of this world . . . even as confused, feverish and mixed-up as it is today! Where there is vigorous health, there is not even an awareness of the complex mechanisms and chemistry that go on inside of us to make this possible. Within our bodies, the most magnificent chemical and mechanical procedures known and unknown to man are carried on.

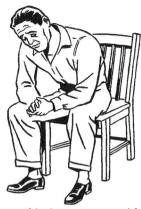

This is a person with chronic fatigue. He has no energy, vitality, strength or ambition. He suffers from extreme weariness physically and mentally, which is a very toxic state of physical deterioration.

We take our health for granted, as we do the moon and the sun – usually even neglecting to be thankful. We get up in the morning after a sound night's sleep, ready to take on the day's work and expect to end the day comfortably tired. It's best to earn your sleep with work and exercise – then you will sleep better for sure!

Miracle Mechanisms of Your Body

If we had transparent skin and could look inside ourselves, we would see the lungs taking air into their delicately fashioned chambers. If we smoked, we would see tobacco's vicious nicotine and tars coating these pink, beautiful, healthy organs to a sticky, deadly black. **If you smoke – stop now! The strong survive longer!**

We would see the heart receiving blood through numerous intricate channels from the billions of our body's cells and pumping it out, refreshed and purified, by another route back to these same tissues. We would get an exact picture of our arteries, veins and capillaries. We could see how much corrosion is taking place because of our consumption of the heavy inorganic minerals and toxic chemicals that are put into our drinking water. If we could examine our arteries closely, we would see that calcium carbonate and its associates are lining these pipes and making them brittle – beginning to literally turn our bodies into stone. Oh, if everyone could see what inorganic minerals do to the arteries – they would be sure to follow the wise advice given in this book! Remember, we are as young as our arteries!

If we could look inside ourselves, we would also see the digestive tract performing miraculous changes to the foods and drinks we consume. We would 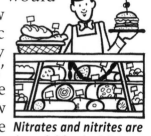 see our body transform salads, raw nuts, seeds, raw and cooked organic vegetables, fruits and other healthy foods into vital substances our bodies' cells need and use! People who live on devitalized diets would see how the body's chemistry labors to handle burgers, hot dogs, processed deli meats,

Nitrates and nitrites are harmful food additives.

high fat and sugar foods, ice cream, candy, colas and all other "fast food trash" that insults, sickens and clogs their digestive tracts and bodies!

If we could get a full view of the largest organ in the body, the liver, we would see how it struggles to handle alcohol, coffee, tea, cola, soft drinks and other unhealthy liquids. We would see the disastrous effects of the dangerous inorganic chemicals that are added to our drinking water by man. Mother Nature can also often do more harm than man by contaminating water with inorganic mineral carbonates and many other substances. Looking closely, we would see that the liver is slowly hardening into stone.

Thousands of people die from a disease known as cirrhosis of the liver – fibrosis, which is a hardening caused by excessive formation of connective tissue followed by contraction of the liver. Both hard water's inorganic minerals and alcohol consumption hardens the liver! Humans recklessly consuming toxic alcohol products is leading to grave health problems! Please drinkers, beware and stop (see web: *www.aa.org*).

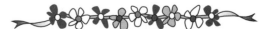

Up to 90% of deaths annually are self-inflicted by an unhealthy lifestyle!

Good health and good sense are two of life's greatest blessings.
– Publilius Syrus, 1st Century B.C.

Hardening of the Arteries is Deadly

On several occasions during my father's boyhood his parents took him to the famous Luray Limestone Caverns in Virginia. There he saw how, drop by drop, water loaded with limestone slowly formed the stalactites and stalagmites over eons of time. These were huge formations created by deposits of the inorganic minerals that are ever-present unfortunately even in most drinking water.

Calcium carbonate, or lime, is a very important and needed ingredient in making cement or concrete. This catalytic agent is responsible for the hardening of concrete. When taken into the body chemistry and subjected to the process of natural metabolism through the years, this mineral becomes the principal troublemaker responsible for what is called "hardening of the arteries." Doctors call this degenerative arterial condition "arteriosclerosis," and most people believe it to be a natural condition that comes with the passing of the years. This is "herd mentality" thinking – or rather, non-thinking! Very few people question this age-old superstition. Many people accept the fallacy that they must face arteriosclerosis and senility in their golden years. Read on – be informed.

Most doctors assert that there is no known cure when hardening of the arteries takes place. New techniques have been developed to implant plastic arteries in place of the clogged arteries and veins of the heart and neck. There are expensive heart vascular surgeries and other expensive surgical procedures for cleaning out the inorganic deposits of the larger arteries (the U.S. spends over $150 billion yearly to try to remedy the affects of bad diet). But when you consider the extent of the entire pipe system of the human body, cleaning out a small amount could not accomplish a great deal. Miles of arteries, veins and capillaries would have to be cleansed of their inorganic crust to be effective. Read on for solutions to stop this hardening by living The Bragg Healthy Lifestyle, to keep your heart and body healthy!

 The body's need for minerals is largely met through foods, not drinking water. – American Medical Association

A man is as old as his arteries – his river of life. – Rudolph Virchow

Normal Artery Compared to Clogged Artery

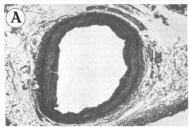 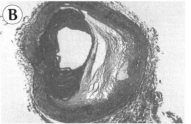

Healthy Open Artery   Cholesterol Clogged Artery

These photomicrographs show (A) a normal artery seen in cross section and (B) a diseased artery in which the channel is partially occluded by atherosclerosis.

Brains Turned to Stone

The greatest damage done by inorganic minerals – plus waxy cholesterol and salt (sodium chloride) – is to the small arteries and other blood vessels of the brain. It also causes deterioration of the kidneys, liver, heart and other vital organs of the body. Essentially, premature ageing and senility are the brain turning into stone! Visit convalescent and rest homes and see with your own eyes the number of people who can no longer reason or think for themselves. Many of them cannot even recognize their own children and relatives!

Millions of people have lost all power of thinking! They often have no control over their eliminative organs and have to wear diapers. Many of them have to be hand fed. All higher functions of the brain and nerves are gone. Their minds and eyes sadly stare into empty space.

This is the way many end up! Millions are saved from this tragedy because they die before their body chemistry has time to turn their brains to stone. Hardening of the arteries and calcification of the blood vessels starts the day you are born, because from birth we begin taking in inorganic minerals and chemicals into our bodies.

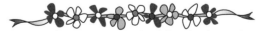

No power on earth can restore the life of a brain hardened by inorganic minerals that has virtually turned to stone.

 Your life will improve, glow and sparkle with health, when you follow The Bragg Healthy Lifestyle!!! – Patricia Bragg

Miracle Functions of the Human Brain

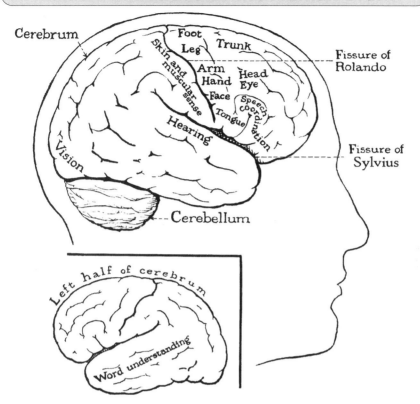

Your Brain Needs Life-Giving Oxygen

Our neighbor, James K., is 65 years old. You will note that we said 65 years *old*, unfortunately not 65 years young. Jim will be forced to retire from his position as an executive in a large company in a few months!

Why do so many large corporations require all employees to retire at age 65? The main reason is that by age 65, most people have hardening of the arteries of the brain. The brain has lost much of its blood supply and is not getting the life-giving oxygen that it needs to keep it healthy, sharp, creative, wide-awake and positive.

Remember that many of the capillaries supplying the brain are as small as a human hair. Years of drinking chemicalized, inorganic mineral water and years of eating a highly unbalanced diet heavy in salt have created masses of toxic acid crystals! These crystals harden the arteries, veins and capillaries that must supply the brain with the needed blood for full brain power!

The Nervous System is the Communication Network of the Body

There is a definite strong link between physical vigor and mental vigor. It all comes down to the fact that we must have a sound mind in a healthy body.

Some people actually build rock formations in their blood vessels supplying blood to their brains, just as great rock formations are made slowly in limestone caverns. You can see how these great columns of stalactites and stalagmites are formed, one drop at a time by inorganic mineral water. The brain does not turn into stone in a few years. But year after year of ingesting inorganic mineral water and toxic foods will slowly build these rock formations in your brain and throughout your body!

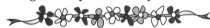

The nervous system, which is made up of the brain and nerves, is the communication system of the body. Note that the nerves vary considerably in diameter and length.

The nervous system consists of two sections controlled by a centralized *"computer"* command center – the brain:

1. External Nervous System: controls the skin surface and external muscles of the body. It transmits to the brain's command center that governs movements of the arms, legs, head and other external muscles, as well as the skin's sensitivity to heat, cold and injury.

2. Internal Nervous System: known as the Autonomic System – it has two subsystems, the Sympathetic and the Parasympathetic (see chart next page). These govern the internal functions of the body (i.e., the vital organs).

The nervous system suffers and falters when we do not take care of our body.

Mother Nature and its beauty is the signature of God. – Patricia Bragg.

Autonomic Nervous System
– The Body's Communication Network –

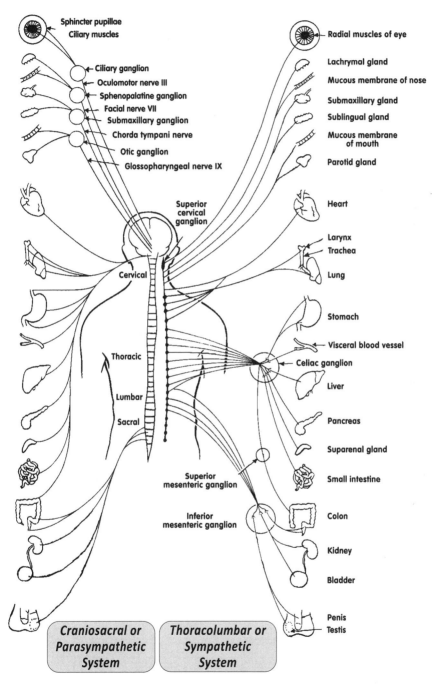

Sphincter pupillae
Ciliary muscles

Radial muscles of eye

Ciliary ganglion
Oculomotor nerve III
Sphenopalatine ganglion
Facial nerve VII
Submaxillary ganglion
Chorda tympani nerve
Otic ganglion
Glossopharyngeal nerve IX

Lachrymal gland
Mucous membrane of nose
Submaxillary gland
Sublingual gland
Mucous membrane of mouth
Parotid gland

Superior cervical ganglion

Heart

Cervical

Larynx
Trachea
Lung

Stomach

Visceral blood vessel
Celiac ganglion

Thoracic

Liver

Lumbar

Pancreas

Sacral

Suparenal gland

Superior mesenteric ganglion

Small intestine

Inferior mesenteric ganglion

Colon

Kidney

Bladder

Penis
Testis

Craniosacral or Parasympathetic System

Thoracolumbar or Sympathetic System

47

Autonomic Nervous System, showing its 2 divisions:
the Craniosacral or Parasympathetic System, and
the Thoracolumbar or Sympathetic System.

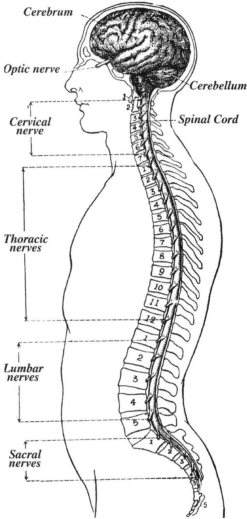

Cerebrum

Optic nerve

Cervical nerve

Thoracic nerves

Lumbar nerves

Sacral nerves

Cerebellum

Spinal Cord

48

It is in the cushions between the bones of the spine that inorganic minerals from water may deposit themselves. This buildup can cause painful stiffness, backaches, slipped discs and many other spinal-back problems. Important Nerve Force to the vital organs may then be greatly reduced, causing painful miseries throughout the entire body.

Studies show drinking 8 glasses of pure distilled water can help ease or even eliminate back and joint pain for up to 80% of sufferers.

I have found distilled water is a sovereign remedy for my rheumatism. I attribute my perfect health largely to distilled water.
– Dr. Alexander Graham Bell, Inventor of the Telephone

8-10 Glasses Purified Water Daily Promotes Super Health and Also Healthy Elimination!

Colon cleanliness is important for superior health! See that your daily liquid intake is at least 8 glasses of distilled/purified water, plus some apple cider vinegar drinks (see recipe page 130) and vegetable or fruit juices, especially if bowel movements are dry. Many people suffer from constipation and hemorrhoids due to dehydration because they don't drink enough water! Remember salt, black tea, coffee, alcohol and soft drinks are dehydrating! One function of the lower bowel is to remove surplus water from the waste. If wastes are not evacuated or remain in the colon too long and a great deal of water is removed, then the stools become too hard to easily eliminate. These poisons must be moved out of the body – no meal should stay in the colon more than 36 hours. When the normal rhythm of bowel evacuation is reached, many of your physical problems will vanish! Read more on page 117.

The Digestive System

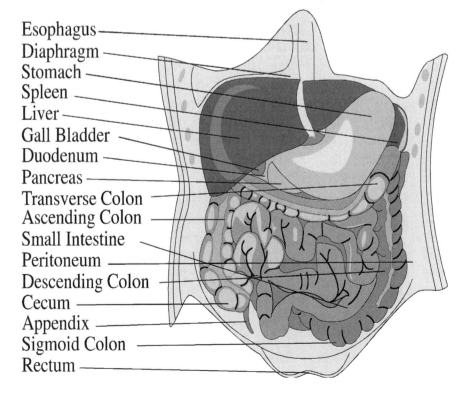

Esophagus

Diaphragm

Stomach

Spleen

Liver

Gall Bladder

Duodenum

Pancreas

Transverse Colon

Ascending Colon

Small Intestine

Peritoneum

Descending Colon

Cecum

Appendix

Sigmoid Colon

Rectum

The Parade of the "Living Dead"

Just remember that physically, chemically and mentally we are what we eat and drink! Because most humans are ignorant about what to put into their bodies, very few escape being one of the *"living dead."* So many people, after their 20s, do not know what healthy, vibrant, youthful living is! They drag themselves through life, relying on some kind of medication to keep them going. They need a "pep" pill to keep them going during the day and a sleeping pill to put them to sleep at night.

How Drinking Water Affects Your Health

Pure water is a necessity for health! In research begun back in the 1960's, the water supply of 1,633 of the largest cities in the U.S. was analyzed. The shocking results of this long study showed a definite link between water quality and the mortality rate from cancer, cardiovascular disease, birth defects and other chronic diseases.

Total Dissolved Solids and Chronic Disease

In his study, "Relationship of Water to the Risk of Dying," Dr. Sauer chronicled the relationship of *Total Dissolved Solids* to heart disease, cancer and other chronic diseases (*Total Dissolved Solids* – or TDS – is the term for all the elements present in any water supply). It had been thought for centuries that the European mineral waters so very high in TDS were beneficial to health. But Dr. Sauer's study found that as TDS increases in a water supply, so does the number of chronic diseases in the population using that water.

(Author's Note: At our home in Desert Hot Springs, one of California's renowned hot mineral water resorts, our corroded water pipes had to be replaced after only a few years due to inorganic mineral buildup in the pipes. What this inorganic mineral-laced water does to plumbing in homes – it also does to the human pipes!)

When our cells are not fully hydrated, they cannot function at optimal levels and this leads to ageing. – Dr. Howard Murad

High Blood Pressure and Drinking Water

Water quality also plays a part in the development of hypertension, or high blood pressure. Hypertension afflicts over 50 million people in the U.S., making it the most common chronic disease. It is also a major health problem in all of the developed countries of the world – due to stress, introduction of refined foods, soft drinks, salt, lack of exercise, and water dehydration.

But the good news about hypertension, or high blood pressure, is that it can be reduced or even prevented! A diet high in natural fiber, grains, vegetables, organic calcium and potassium – with less meat, fat and sodium, can help reduce or even prevent hypertension.

It's estimated that over 10% of our sodium intake is from drinking water! A study of high school sophomores in a community with high levels of sodium in their drinking water showed significantly higher blood pressure levels than those in areas with less sodium in their water. The girls among this first group had blood pressure patterns characteristic of persons 10 years older! Follow up studies in the same area among even younger children, ages 7 to 11 years, produced similar results.

51

The conclusion from this and other studies seems obvious: increased sodium levels in drinking water leads to increased blood pressure levels. The American Heart Association, the EPA (Environmental Protection Agency) and the World Health Organization – among other health groups – recommend that sodium levels in drinking water should not exceed 20 mg/liter! And yet, of 2,100 water companies included in a survey by the U.S. Public Health Service, 42% had sodium ion concentrations above this so called safe level! About 5% showed shocking levels greater than 250 mg/liter!

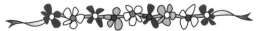

Daily use of distilled water is a marvelous blood purifier, diluting toxins in the body as well as aiding in their elimination through the kidneys. It should be used for cooking, baking & drinking. – Dr. Charles McFerrin, "Nature's Path", 1955

 Distilled water helps keep your heart, lungs, brain, liver, and skin healthy and vital.

Water Softeners Use Sodium = Trouble!

We have already seen the strong relationship between soft water and heart disease! But that is only part of the story – for softened water also poses grave health risks in terms of hypertension (high blood pressure) problems.

The usual method for softening water is to add 2 parts sodium (salt) which then extracts 1 part calcium and 1 part magnesium from the water supply. This results in "softer" water which is higher in sodium, a good reason to avoid water softeners! So it would seem the "luxury" of having soft water to bathe in and for laundry is not worth the increased risks to your health and longevity!

Dangerous Chemicals In Our Drinking Water – Causing Cancer and Heart Disease Epidemics

There is more and more evidence that the majority of human cancers are environmental in origin and thereby largely preventable! In fact, an astounding number of chemical – and possibly carcinogenic – compounds are found in our water supplies after treatment and in surface and ground water sources.

An ABC News exposé revealed the shocking fact that over 700 chemicals have already been found in our drinking water! Of these, 129 have been pinpointed by the EPA as posing serious health risks! Yet that same agency requires that our water supplies be regularly tested for only 14 of the 129 serious health risk chemicals!

One carcinogen found in many municipal water systems, chloroform, can be introduced during chlorine treatment. A known animal carcinogen, it is present in measurable levels in nearly all nation-wide municipal water systems as a by-product of water chlorination!

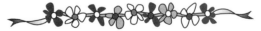

In contemplating the nature of water I feel that it is the mother, the life of all material manifestation. It is the most flexible and yet the most solid, the most destructive but, next to air, the most necessary. No matter how much it is mixed with other substances, when we distill it, it is cleansed and purified into clean distilled water so that we can drink it to our health benefit. – Jeanne Keller, author of "Healing with Water"

The Sad Truth About Chlorination

Water chlorination has been widely used to "purify" water in America since 1904. But its negative effects on health surely outweigh any benefits. Dr. Joseph Price, (see page 55) for one, believes that there is a definite link between widespread chlorination of water supplies and the increasing incidence of heart disease! In the animal experiments he conducted, chlorine caused atherosclerosis in 95% of the animals tested! Chlorine in the water supply has been linked with cancers of the bladder, liver, pancreas and urinary tract in certain areas. To take just one example of what is happening around the world, in New Orleans the drinking water is taken from the Mississippi River. Over 66 new carcinogenic compounds have been isolated in that city's water supply as a result of adding chlorine – a substance which naturally combines with methanol, carbon disulfide and other compounds! A very high incidence of colon cancer has been found in this city and surrounding areas.

Cancers and Chlorination

An investigator at the government's National Cancer Institute, Kenneth Cantor, points out that many studies even since the early 1974 report on New Orleans have confirmed its findings, linking increased carcinogens in the water supply to additional cancer deaths annually. Cantor and his associates completed a study of nearly 3,000 men and women who had been drinking chlorinated water in cities such as New York, Chicago, Atlanta, Detroit, New Orleans, San Francisco and Seattle. Subjects were also studied in Connecticut, Iowa, New Jersey, New Mexico and Utah. This study conclusively linked bladder cancer to drinking chlorinated water!

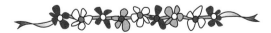

Ample evidence points to chlorine-based chemicals as significant contributors to breast cancer. – Joe Thornton, author of
- *"Breast Cancer and The Environment: The Chlorine Connection"*
- *"Pandora's Poison: Chlorine, Health & A New Environmental Strategy"*

Wisdom is found only in truth. – Johann Wolfgang von Goethe

Nor is the risk limited to just bladder cancer alone. Theresa Young of the Department of Preventive Medicine at the University of Wisconsin led a revealing study to determine the effect of chlorinated water on women. She checked death certificates of women in Wisconsin who had died from cancers of the gastrointestinal system, the urinary tract, the brain, lungs and breast.

The major finding was that colon cancer in women was "significantly associated" with exposure to water which was disinfected with low, medium and high daily chlorine doses for at least 20 years! She stated that researchers should pursue other theories of colon cancer as well – such as industrial pollutants and chlorine-induced carcinogens in drinking water. She also said her study should be examined in the context of the theory linking colon cancer to a high fat, low fiber diet.

One expert, Dr. Herbert Schwartz, states emphatically that "chlorine is so dangerous it should be banned!" He believes that chlorine-treated water alone is directly responsible for cancer, heart disease and premature senility growth! See web: *www.ZeroWasteAmerica.org*

54

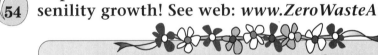

"Your Body's Many Cries for Water; You're Not Sick, You're Thirsty, Don't Treat Thirst with Medication"

These are powerful quotes from F. Batmanghelidj, M.D.'s book

- *Pure water is a natural medication for a variety of health conditions.*
- *Chronic cellular dehydration can painfully and prematurely kill. Its initial outward manifestations have until now unfortunately been erroneously labeled as diseases of unknown origin.*
- *For process of food digestion, water is the most essential ingredient. If the body has the necessary water in it before we eat food, the battle against cholesterol formation in the blood vessels might be won.*
- *Cholesterol production in the cell membrane is a part of the cell survival system. It is a necessary substance. Its excess denotes dehydration.*
- *Dehydration causes stress, and stress will cause further dehydration.*
- *Pure water is the cheapest form of medicine to a dehydrated body!*
  Visit Dr. Batmanghelidj's website: www.WaterCure.com

The kind of water you drink can make or break you – your body is 75% water!

Chlorine Chemical Cocktail is Deadly

Dr. Joseph Price, famous U.S. medical researcher and author of *Coronaries/Cholesterol/Chlorine* stated, "Chlorine is the greatest crippler and killer of modern times. Two decades after the start of chlorination of our drinking water system in 1904, the present epidemic of heart disease and cancer began." (Still epidemic now in the 21st Century.)

Can Miscarriages and Birth Defects Be Caused by Chlorinated Tap Water?

The Environmental Working Group and U.S. Public Interest Research Group admit that adding chlorine to tap water saves thousands of lives each year by reducing the number of harmful bacteria. However, they say that this process itself actually creates **hundreds of toxic chemicals called "chlorination by-products," or** CBPs.

Many cities large and small have reported potentially dangerous levels of CBPs in their tap water over the past six years, according to the report. In total, the investigators list 42 cities – both large and small – that expose pregnant women each year to trihalomethanes (THM), the most common toxic chlorination by-product.

A standard by the Environmental Protection Agency in effect lowers the allowed levels of chlorination by-products, including THMs. However, the investigators list multiple cities with lower levels of THM in tap water that they say still expose thousands of women to potentially serious and dangerous toxins during their pregnancy!!!

"It's not a big surprise," says Joel Schwartz, Ph.D., Associate Professor of Environmental Epidemiology, Harvard School of Public Health. Dr. Schwartz says recent studies have linked toxic chlorine by-products to reproduction risks! In other studies his group found CBPs could affect a baby's birth weight and pointed to risks of dangerous birth defects and miscarriage. – *webmd.com*

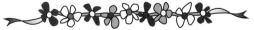

Drinking water disinfected by chlorine while pregnant may increase the risk of having children with heart problems, cleft palate or major brain defects, according to study published in Environmental Health Journal.
– ScienceDaily.com

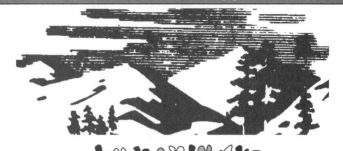

Ten Tips for Good Health

- *Respect and protect your body as the highest manifestation of your life.*

- *Abstain from unnatural, devitalized foods and stimulating beverages.*

- *Nourish your body with only natural unprocessed, live foods.*

- *Extend your years in health for loving, sharing and charitable service.*

- *Regenerate your body by the right balance of activity and rest.*

- *Purify your cells, tissue and blood with healthy organic foods, and*
  with pure water, clean air and gentle sunshine.

- *Abstain from all food when out of sorts in mind or body.*

- *Keep thoughts, words and emotions pure, calm, loving and uplifting.*

- *Increase your knowledge of Mother Nature's Laws, follow them,*
  and enjoy the fruits of your life's labor.

- *Lift up yourself, friends and family by loyal obedience to*
  Mother Nature's and God's Healthy, Natural Laws of Living.

Patricia Bragg and *Paul C. Bragg*

Bragg Healthy Lifestyle Plan

- *Read, plan, plot, and follow through for supreme health and longevity.*
- *Underline, highlight or dog-ear pages as you read important passages.*
- *Organizing your lifestyle helps you identify what's important in your life.*
- *Be faithful to your health goals daily for a healthy, long, fulfilled life.*
- *Where space allows we have included "words of wisdom" from great minds*
  to motivate and inspire you. Please share your favorite sayings with us.
- *Write us about your successes following The Bragg Healthy Lifestyle.*

Open your eyes so you may behold wondrous things out of Thy law.
– Psalm 119:18

Chapter 5

The Paul C. Bragg Story

Paul C. Bragg's Early Experiences With Hard Water

Where I was raised we got our drinking water from a well overflowing with crystalline, fresh water. It was very hard water because it contained a great deal of calcium carbonate and other inorganic minerals from limestone in suspension or solution.

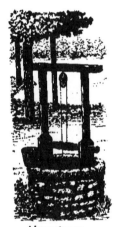

This hard water made laundering and cleaning difficult. The soap used for these purposes simply would not make suds.

When we boiled this water, inorganic mineral encrustations formed in large slabs inside the kettles. In time, it created holes in the bottoms of the kettles. Kettle after kettle had to be thrown away, with the same deteriorations happening to each kettle!

But the greatest damage done to humans who drank this hard, inorganic mineral water was to their entire cardiovascular systems and their overall health.

Limestone Water

57

My grandfather was a man in his mid-sixties. He was a big, strong six-footer – about 200 pounds of solid muscle. My grandfather was a loving Christian family man, an expert horseman and a hard working farmer.

I can remember when my grandfather had his first stroke. There was a large family gathering of Braggs, and we were all seated together around the Sunday dinner table. Suddenly, there was a loud crash of dishes when grandfather slumped over the table. When the country doctor arrived, he stated sadly that grandfather

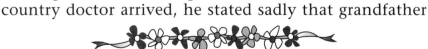

Teach me Thy way O Lord; and lead me in a plain path. – Psalms 27:11

had lost all control of his left side due to the brain damage from a stroke. From then on, he needed constant attention. With a completely paralyzed left side, he could not walk without the aid of someone to steady him. He had absolutely no control of his eliminative system. There was great difficulty getting food into his body because he had lost the ability to chew. We could only feed him very soft, mashed foods, vegetables, potatoes, fruits and soups.

This fine man we knew and loved was, as far as real living was concerned, dead. You have no idea what a great burden he was on my parents and family. The poor, helpless man struggled on in this manner for 3 years. Then the second and final stroke came and he died. The doctors who performed the autopsy stated that his arteries were like stone. My grandfather was born and reared on that farm and drank that hard water every day and he paid for it with his life.

Discovered Miseries Caused by Hard Water

I was just a little boy when my father explained to me the outcome of my grandfather's autopsy. I asked my father in despair, "How could his arteries turn into stone?" He couldn't give a satisfactory answer to my question. That very day, I resolved to find out why my grandfather's arteries had hardened.

I read medical books loaned to me by my Uncle William, who was our family doctor. I besieged my uncle with hundreds of questions as to why human arteries could become like stone. It was to be many years before my questions were answered. Over time, I witnessed what hard water was doing to my family, our relatives and friends. It also corroded our water pipes (page 50).

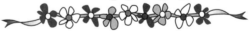

Eminent physicians for years have recognized and advocated the health value of distilled water, both for prevention of disease and for restoration of health. It tends to ward off the ageing process by preventing the formation of calcareous deposits that cause hardening of the arteries.
– C.W. DeLacy Evans, M.D., author "How to Prolong Life"

Drinking the right water in the right quantity at the right time is just as important as eating well. Pure distilled water is the right drink!
– Paul C. Bragg, N.D., Ph.D., Originator of Health Stores

Millions Suffer With Joint Pain

One of the women who worked in our home was named Bessie Louise. She was just like a member of the family, and we all loved her dearly. Poor Bessie developed arthritis and rheumatism in her hands, wrists, elbows, hips, knees and ankles. How that poor woman suffered day after day from tormenting pain! Sometimes the pain would be so great that she would burst into tears.

Again I asked my Uncle William, what caused the arthritis. I wanted to know if there was a cure for this tormenting condition. He answered me honestly. "Paul," Uncle William said, "we do not know the cause of crippling, painful arthritis, and we have no cure for it. All I can do is give Bessie strong painkillers to relieve her great pain and suffering."

SEVEN TYPES OF JOINTS

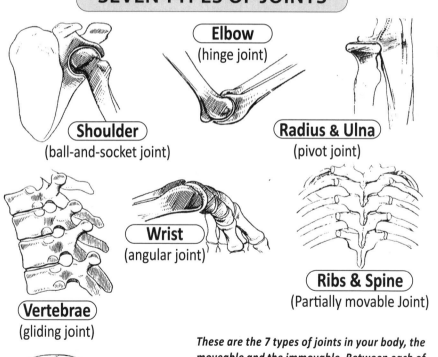

Elbow
(hinge joint)

Shoulder
(ball-and-socket joint)

Radius & Ulna
(pivot joint)

Wrist
(angular joint)

Ribs & Spine
(Partially movable Joint)

Vertebrae
(gliding joint)

Cranium
(immovable joint)

These are the 7 types of joints in your body, the moveable and the immovable. Between each of the moveable joints there is a clear amber fluid called synovial fluid which acts as a lubricant to keep the joints moving freely and easily. When inorganic minerals from drinking water and toxic acid crystals replace this synovial fluid you experience stiffness, pain and misery.

In time, poor Bessie was confined to her bed in pain. In just a few years she was dead. She never reached 65. Sadly her last years were filled with intense pain, misery and suffering.

My poor young brain suffered. "What causes this horrible, crippling disease?" I would ask myself in the late hours before going to sleep.

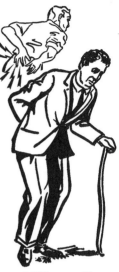

Here we were living with an abundant supply of foods of all kinds. We had a good, comfortable home. But there was suffering among the adults. These pains were grouped under one word, and that was "misery"! Each day I would hear my mother ask different people, "How

Millions suffer with joint pain.

is your misery today?" The sufferers would answer my mother dolefully.

Frustrated, I would go to our kind and patient doctor, Uncle William, and put the question squarely to him. "Uncle," I would ask, "Why do so many people suffer from the misery?" His answer was, "I wish I knew." Then again I would say to myself, "Someday, I will find out why people suffer from the *misery*"!

T.B. in My Teens – Changed and Guided My Life! and My Future!

When I was just a lad I saved a man from drowning. As it turns out this man was very rich and to reward me for saving his life he gave me a scholarship to a large military school. My parents were very eager for me to attend, so at the tender age of 12, I was enrolled in a large military school in the south. At the military school, I not only drank hard water, but I was fed a poor institutional diet. We were served loads of starches such as refined flour hot cakes, biscuits and white rice. For our meals, we could

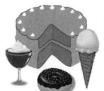

select several overcooked meats, hot dogs, sausages, fried potatoes, and end up with heavy desserts loaded with white sugar including doughnuts, sweet buns, candy, chocolate cakes, pies, cookies, puddings, and ice cream.

In four years, at only age 16, I was a sad victim of tuberculosis. Again and again I asked my uncle who was a doctor why this had happened to me. He could not answer my question.

I spent time in several T.B. Sanitariums – to no avail – and then fate intervened. I was skin and bones and so sick and weak! When four staff doctors examined me, I asked them point-blank, "Are you going to save me from this disease?" I received an honest answer. "No," they said, "We don't believe you're going to make it."

When they left the room, my human angel – Maria, the Swiss exchange nurse – seemed angry. "These American doctors know nothing about T.B.," she declared. "I am glad I am returning to a Sanitarium and a doctor who has cures!" I cried out, "Will you take me to that doctor? I want to live so I may help all sick people!"

I Want To Be A Health Crusader!

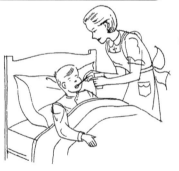

So, the Swiss nurse took me to her wonderful Sanitarium in Switzerland where the great physician, Dr. August Rollier, gave me a new life by using all natural healing methods. He administered no drugs of any kind – just distilled (rain) water, good nutrition, sunshine, fresh air, deep breathing, massage and exercise. In 2 years, I was healthy and strong as a young stallion. Now I was ready to achieve my life's ambition of helping others to help themselves to superb health!

61

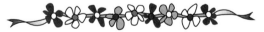

Dear friend, I wish above all things that thou may prosper and be in health even as the soul prospers. – 3 John 2

 Nature, time and patience are the three greatest physicians. – Irish Proverb

---

Let nature be your teacher. – William Wordsworth

Seek and find the best for your body, mind and soul. – Patricia Bragg

Calcium & Magnesium are especially important for healthy bones & heart.

Locations in the Body Where Osteoporosis, Arthritis, Pain and Misery Hit the Hardest

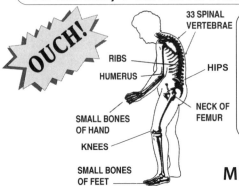

OSTEOPOROSIS
Affects over 60 Million and Kills 400,000 Americans Annually
Estimated 50% of adults 65 years or older also suffer from Arthritis.

Boron: Miracle Trace Mineral For Healthy Bones

BORON – An important trace mineral for healthier and stronger bones that also helps the body absorb more vital calcium, minerals and necessary hormones! Good boron sources are most organic veggies, fresh and sun-dried fruits, avocados, prunes, and raw nuts.

The U.S. Dept. of Agriculture's Nutrition Lab in Grand Forks, ND, says Boron is usually found in soil and foods, but many Americans eat a diet low in Boron. They conducted a 17 week study which showed a daily 3 to 6 mgs. Boron supplement enabled participants to reduce loss (demineralization) of calcium, phosphorus and magnesium from their bodies. This loss is usually caused by eating processed fast foods, drinking tap waters (distilled is best), eating lots of meat, salt, sugar and fat and a dietary lack of fresh vegetables, fruits and whole grains. (*all-natural.com*)

Scientific studies show women benefit from a healthy lifestyle that includes vitamin D3 sunshine and exercise (even weight-lifting) to maintain healthier bones, combined with distilled water, low-fat, high-fiber, carbohydrates, and fresh organic fruits, salads, sprouts, greens and vegetable diet. This lifestyle helps protect against heart disease, high blood pressure, cancer and many other ailments! I'm happy to see science now agrees with my Dad who first stated these health truths in the 1920's.

For more hormone and osteoporosis facts read pioneer Dr. John R. Lee's book – "What Your Doctor May Not Tell You About Menopause"

Boron helps keep skeletal structure strong by adding to bone density, preventing Osteoporosis, treating Arthritis and improving strength and muscle mass. Boron helps facilitate calcium directly into the bones. Boron protects bones by regulating Estrogen function. Boron is naturally found in beans, nuts, avocados, berries, plums, oranges and grapes. Boron helps relieve menopause symptoms and PMS. – Dr. Axe

The Secret of Rain and Snow Water: It's Distilled By Mother Nature

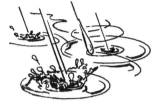

Many of Dr. Rollier's Sanitarium practices are now standard T.B. treatment. In many ways, this doctor was years ahead of others and his wise health care saved my life!

He was very insistent upon one point: "No hard water should ever be given to a patient." Although water is abundant in Switzerland, Dr. Rollier gave us only water from clean rain and melted snow (distilled by Mother Nature). He was also a great believer in the use of fresh vegetable and fruit juices. Dr. Rollier always told us the reasons for his treatments. He explained, "Practically all of the water in Switzerland is *heavy* or *hard* water, loaded with inorganic minerals. This hard water burdens and brings only harm to our bodies, because the body chemistry can assimilate only organic living foods and liquids."

I admired, loved and followed Dr. Rollier because he gave logical answers to my questions. What a brilliant man! He brought healing to patients from all over the world who had been doomed to die, including myself. When I left the sanitarium, he cautioned me that I must drink only rain and snow waters, vegetable and fruit juices (all distilled by Mother Nature) and distilled water.

The Answer to Healthful Living

Pondering Dr. Rollier's advice, I thought, "Could it be possible my grandfather's death from a stroke and Bessie Louise's death from crippling arthritis had a common basis? Was it due to drinking hard water and eating devitalized foods?" These questions nagged at me. I felt a great burden that could be lifted only when I found the answers.

"Water hardness (inorganic minerals in solution) is the underlying cause of many, if not all, of the diseases resulting from poisons in the intestinal tract. These (hard minerals) pass from the intestinal walls and get into the lymphatic system, which delivers all of its products to the blood, which in turn, distributes to all parts of the body. This is the cause of much human disease." —Dr. Charles Mayo of the Mayo Clinic

Inspired to learn and research natural healing methods, we've in turn been blessed by helping millions to better health and remain enthusiastic about the miracle healing powers of God and Mother Nature. That's why we wrote this life-changing book, which has lead the way to pure water for millions. Here are the answers that may help save millions from suffering!

My First Challenging Case - The Wilsons

As noted earlier, after my two years at Dr. Rollier's Sanitarium in Switzerland, I was reborn with a new healthy life! Completely cured of T.B., I was in excellent condition. The Alpine sunshine, the pure rain and snow distilled water to drink, the clean air of the Alps and the natural diet had given me a new body. Every cell in my body vibrated with vigorous health! Now I was ready to study biochemistry and other related health subjects to prepare for my life's work being a Health Crusader.

Deciding to live and study in London, I found a small apartment not far from the famous Regent's Park. In my opinion, this is one of the most beautiful parks in the world. Here I could take my early morning runs, and play tennis. In my apartment, I could prepare and enjoy my live food meals and fresh juices.

The owner of the building lived on the first floor. He and his wife were the typical, prematurely old people. They ate the regular English diet. It contained refined white flour (bread, biscuits, pastries and other refined products), large amounts of sugar and jams and jellies along with gallons

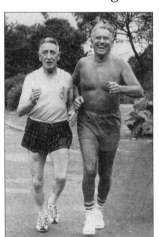

of black tea full of sugar and milk. Their vegetables and meats were all overcooked. To top it all, they drank London tap water, which was heavily chlorinated, chemicalized and loaded with calcium carbonate and harmful toxins that cause stiffness and health problems.

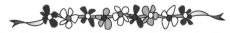

Paul C. Bragg and Duncan McLean, England's oldest champion sprinter (83 years young) on a training run in London's famous Regent's Park.

When I came to inspect the fifth floor apartment – a "walk-up" with no "lift" or elevator – the owner, Mr. Wilson, gave me the key and told me his joints were so stiff that he could not walk up the five flights. So I went up alone and found the apartment to be exactly what I wanted. Among other things to my liking, it was unheated. However, there were small, built-in grates; if I wanted heat, I would have to order coal and have it delivered in bags, so I could carry it upstairs.

I settled down comfortably in my fifth floor London apartment and started my schooling in biochemistry. My landlords, the Wilsons, were very friendly and from time to time I would drop by their apartment for a visit. Both of these nice English people had numerous physical troubles. Mr. Wilson suffered greatly from low back pain, as well as pains in all his moveable joints and some form of bladder disease. Mrs. Wilson was not much better off. She was 50 pounds overweight and huffed and puffed with every move. She also suffered from kidney disease. During my visits, a good part of our conversation was centered around their many body ailments.

By this time, the cruel London winter had set in. Outside, it was damp and cold. But each day before dawn, I would put on my heavy sweat clothes and take a long run in Regent's Park, returning to the apartment glowing with good circulation and health! I never had as much as a sniffle all winter, but the Wilsons were plagued with one cold after another. They had large amounts of toxic mucus pouring out of them and felt sick most of the winter.

One Saturday, when I stopped by their apartment after my long morning run, I could see that Mr. Wilson was desperately ill. He was running a high fever and his nose was so completely stuffed up that he had to breathe through his mouth. I went into his bedroom, which was overheated and had very little oxygen. The poor man looked up and said, "For God's sake, you're studying health, help me! I feel so sick – like I'm dying!" "Mr. Wilson," I told him confidently, "if you will follow this natural system of healing I outline for you, you can get well!"

Knowing these teachings will mean true life and good health for you.
– Proverbs 4:22

From Sickness to Superb Health

I knew I could help him, but I wondered before making my offer if he was strong enough of mind and wanted to achieve *health* passionately enough? "I will follow your instructions to the letter," he stated in desperation, like a drowning man grasping a helping hand.

"Good! Today you will start on a 10 day cleansing fast." I picked up the bottles on the bedside table. "Soon all this medication will go down the drain." I brought him some of my distilled water, purchased apple cider vinegar, lemons and honey and started him on his first fast day. It was not easy for this man to fast. Mr. Wilson was so full of toxic poisons, so full of sticky mucus in his head, throat and lungs that he had a great deal of discomfort and trouble getting rid of it. But he was an Englishman with plenty of fortitude. He passed a lot of toxic wastes from his sick body. At the end of the 10 day fast, he felt better than he had for years!

Then, I put him on a natural live food diet consisting of fresh fruit and vegetable juices and distilled water. Within 3 weeks after his fast, he climbed the 5 flights of stairs to my apartment – something he had not done in 7 years! His wife became enthusiastic about my natural way of living and began to follow the program which became The Bragg Healthy Lifestyle. She started to shed the fat from her body that she couldn't lose before.

After 6 months you could not tell the Wilsons were the same people. They were healthier, stronger and happier! Mr. Wilson ran up to my apartment twice a day. Now Mrs. Wilson looked trim and slim and had to have all her clothes taken in. Their married daughter lived in Canada and came to visit. She could not believe what she saw.

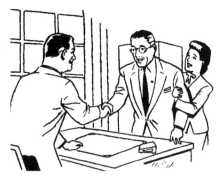

The Wilsons thanked me and said they felt "reborn." By following The Bragg Healthy Lifestyle, they found new, vigorous super health!

Secret of longevity is eating & drinking intelligently. – Gayelord Hauser

The Wilsons' health troubles were gone. They were now enjoying life fully and it made me so happy!

This was my first case – the Wilsons who followed my Bragg Healthy Lifestyle. The results gave me confidence which grew as I studied the teachings of the world's great healers. It was Hippocrates, the Father of Medicine, in 400 B.C. who gave these wise words to the world to use:

Let food be your medicine and medicine be your food.

Mother Nature and God's Way

We give thanks for the millions of people who read Bragg books and have come to us for advice through the years and have been reborn healthy again by living The Bragg Healthy Lifestyle which is God and Mother Nature's Way! We feel blessed to know we've inspired people to make healthy changes in their lives!

This is Mother Nature's own natural lifestyle. There is a big difference between feeling well enough to carry on one's daily activities with no sensation of anything wrong, and that more exhilarating state of health which fills one with enthusiasm for life and its challenges. An adequate amount of that important commodity – vibrant health – supplies sufficient energy for life to go on serenely, but it takes more to give one a sense of exuberance. People who live by Mother Nature's Eternal Laws may enjoy an exalted feeling of well-being that is not euphoric but is rather the result of a natural *joie de vivre* or radiant joy of living.

The Wilsons discovered this joy of living when they changed from their unhealthy lifestyle and tried The Bragg Healthy Lifestyle. They learned through their own experience that the body is a naturally self-repairing and self-healing instrument. Mr. Wilson found out that the stiffness in all his moveable joints was not due to the number of years he had lived, but due to the wrong kinds of food, water and lack of exercise! He learned that time is not toxic, but it's lifestyle and habits that count.

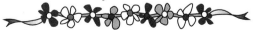

When pure rules of business and conduct are observed, there is true religion. Walk in the path of duty, do good to your brethren and work no evil towards them.

Mr. Wilson's stiffness was brought on by a combination of toxic acid crystals from an unbalanced, acid diet and drinking water saturated with inorganic minerals and toxic chemicals! Fasting helped to dissolve these encrustations which had been deposited in his joints. A natural diet and distilled water continued the cleansing and healing process and helped prevent a recurrence of his former ailments.

The same thing happened with Mrs. Wilson's weight and kidney problems. She felt remarkably improved. By switching from their old unhealthy ways to The Bragg Healthy Lifestyle – Mother Nature's Way – they were able to enjoy their full health potential and experience the true joy of healthy living and superb healthy energy!

The Miracle Life of Jack LaLanne

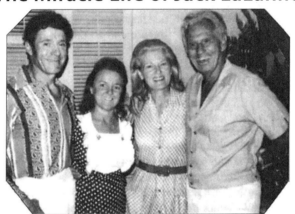

Jack LaLanne, Patricia Bragg, Elaine LaLanne & Paul C. Bragg

Jack says he would have been dead by 16 if he hadn't attended The Bragg Crusade. Jack says, Bragg saved my life at 15, when I attended the Bragg Health Crusade in Oakland, California. From that day, Jack faithfully continued to live The Bragg Healthy Lifestyle, inspiring millions to health, fitness and a long and happy life! See web: *JackLaLanne.com*

To fare well implies the partaking of such food
as does not disagree with body or mind. Hence only those
fare well who live temperately. – Socrates

Perfect Health is above gold; a sound body before riches. – Solomon

Chapter 6

Water and Its Effects On the Human Body

The Stones Within Us

The more we learned about biochemistry (life chemistry), the more we realized why so many people were prematurely old, stiff and suffering from pain throughout their bodies. During our visits to London's largest hospitals, we learned more about stones forming within the human body. Why do stones form in our bodies? What does this mean with regard to our health?

The most common places to find such stones are in the gallbladder, the kidneys, the passageways between kidneys and bladder (known as the ureters) and within the bladder itself. Another organ where stones are sometimes revealed, by an ultrasound, x-ray or CT scan, is the pancreas. This is the glandular organ which lies behind the stomach and has both an internal and an external secretion. Stone formation anywhere in the body has always been regarded as a diseased condition.

69

In our opinion, all these stones are formed by the unbalanced, acid, toxin-producing diet that most humans eat; further aggravated by the chemicalized, inorganically mineralized water they drink. Add to this the heavy concentrations of salt most people use, plus the tremendous amount of waxy cholesterol (saturated fats) ingested by the average person, then unhealthful conditions result! Unbalanced diets form toxic poisons which the body cannot metabolize or easily eliminate, so these toxins are formed into stones by the body's chemistry. Practically all drinking water contains the inorganic mineral calcium carbonate. This and other inorganic minerals and toxins play a big part in the formation of painful stones within the body's organs.

An estimated 37 million adults have kidney disease: Healthy kidneys clean your blood by removing excess fluid, minerals and wastes. But if the kidneys are damaged, they don't work properly. If your kidneys fail, you need treatment to replace the work they normally do. The treatment options are dialysis or kidney transplant. – nlm.nih.gov/medlineplus/kidneyfailure.html

Silent, Painless Gallstones
May Suddenly Become Noisy and Painful

"Silent" gallstones are those which remain quietly in the gallbladder and do not produce the acute abdominal pain which is known as gallstone colic. However, these silent stones may at any time – perhaps at an inopportune moment – become raucously "noisy" and extremely painful!!!

Noisy gallstones may involve not only the gallbladder itself but also the common duct – a vital structure which serves to carry secretions from both the gallbladder and the liver into the intestine. This often happens when the gallbladder contracts and attempts to push out a gallstone. If the stone gets stuck on the way out, there is acute pain, and in many cases, inflammation of the gallbladder and the common duct.

If the stone blocks the common duct, the liver cannot send its bile into the intestine where it is essential for proper and healthy digestion. Then the liver is in trouble! The result is what is known as obstructive jaundice, evidenced by the yellow of the bile which shows up in the skin and in the whites of the eyes.

The color of the skin also betrays the presence of silent gallstones. This was the case with the great Hollywood film actor Tyrone Power, who came to us for some health and diet advise. He looked physically fit, but we could tell from the color of his skin and his eyes that he was suffering with silent gallstones.

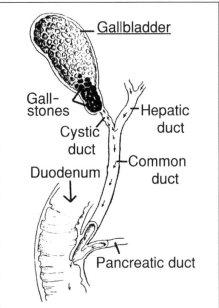

GALLSTONES IN GALLBLADDER
Gallstones may be caused by drinking water saturated with inorganic minerals and deadly toxic crystals formed by an unbalanced, unnatural diet. Also, hardened, saturated fats and hydrogenated foods and their oils can cause some gallbladder problems.

70

We pleaded with him to change his unhealthy habits and follow Mother Nature's way, but sadly we could not get him to change! He died way too young! If he had let us put him on a program of liver and gallbladder detoxification – and given up his unbalanced diet, alcohol, salt and ordinary drinking water – that talented, handsome man may not have had such an early demise!

We have had many people under our nutritional supervision who had gallstones. The following is an excerpt from the Bragg book, *Apple Cider Vinegar – Miracle Health System*. See back pages for booklist.

Apple Cider Vinegar Combats Gallstones

Before starting this two day gallbladder flush, prepare for one week by drinking slowly – upon arising, mid-morning, mid-afternoon and after dinner – $1/2$ tsp. ACV with a 6 oz. glass of apple juice; or if hypoglycemic or diabetic, then dilute with half distilled water. Organic, unfiltered apple juice is rich in malic acid, potassium, pectins and enzymes. These act as solvents to soften and help remove debris (small stones) and cleanse your body. Doctors have non-surgical methods for removing difficult, larger stones using sound waves! But it's best to purge small and medium-sized ones twice yearly as they can grow to cause problems! (See testimony below.)

71

During two-day gallbladder flush no food is eaten, only liquids. Combine in 8 oz glass: $1/3$ cup organic extra-virgin olive oil (no substitutes), $2/3$ cup organic apple juice and 1 tsp. organic ACV with the 'mother.' Drink mixture three times the first day. *At night, sleep on your right side when on flush, pulling right knee toward chest to open pathway.* On second day, take mixture twice. On both days drink all the organic apple juice desired, but no water or any other liquid. (*This gallbladder flush is not for diabetics unless supervised by a health professional.*)

Your book "Apple Cider Vinegar" saved me from having my gallbladder out. The specialist wanted to take my gallbladder out, instead I followed your apple cider vinegar flush and it worked along with healing prayers at church! I think all book and health stores should carry your vinegar book. I am grateful for you writing it. God bless you. – Carmen Puro, Michigan

About midmorning on the third day, eat a raw variety salad (nature's broom) of cabbage, carrots, celery, beets, tomatoes, sprouts and lettuce, with lots of ACV and olive oil. If desired, have a bowl of lightly steamed greens: kale, collards, chard or any leafy greens. Season with ACV and squeeze of lemon – this gives delicious flavor to greens.

We take this miracle cleanser flush at least one or twice a year. Check your bowel movement for tiny, greenish-brown stones. This Flush will amaze you what your gallbladder, stomach and colon will clean out!

Kidney Stones

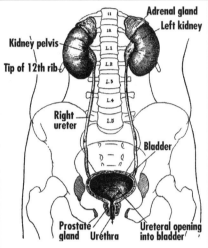

The major cause of most kidney stones is hard, chemicalized water that's saturated heavily with calcium carbonate and other inorganic minerals (read pages 103-106).

Beneath our former home in the California desert, there is a hot subterranean river. When wells are sunk into this river several hundred feet below the earth's surface, the water comes out at 180°F. It's heavily saturated with calcium carbonate and related minerals, such as magnesium carbonate. This water is not channelled through cast iron or steel pipes because costly encrustations of these inorganic minerals will soon block the water flow. Copper pipes are best for hot mineral springs plumbing.

THE URINARY SYSTEM:
Kidneys, Ureters and Bladder

The adrenal glands are shown on top of kidneys. It is in the urinary system that inorganic minerals and toxic acid crystals may cause kidney and bladder stones. The urinary system must be kept free of these deposits to remain in healthy elastic condition characteristic of youthfulness.

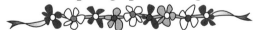

No man can violate Nature's Laws and escape her penalties! – Julian Johnson

Distilled water is the greatest fluid on earth, the only one that can be taken into the body without damage to the tissues.
– Dr. Allen Banik, "The Choice is Clear"

People come from all over the world to bathe in the mineral waters at this spa town. The hot water does have a wonderful curative value. It brings relief to those suffering from arthritis and rheumatism. Most of the hot water pools are kept at a temperature of 104 to 108°F. Our body heat is 98.6°F. When you submerge your body in water hotter than your body temperature, you start an artificial fever and many toxic poisons are eliminated through the 96 million pores of the skin. We all know that a good sweat is refreshing to the body. We always feel lighter after a healthy sweat!

The sad part about coming to the hot water health resort, however, is that people are also advised to drink this water that's heavily saturated by inorganic mineral water, and the high concentrations of these inorganic minerals are extremely dangerous! If you put 5 gallons of this mineral water in a pan and let it evaporate, a slab of hardened inorganic minerals will be left!

Don't Drink Inorganic Mineralized Water

Several years ago, a gentleman from New York came to this hot water resort to take the baths. The uninformed owners of the spa told this man to also drink the mineral water, as it would be good for him. We advised him strongly to bathe only – not to drink the water. But he did not heed our advice. During the 6 months he took the baths, he also drank this water that caused his demise! One night the people in the hotel heard him scream out in agonized pain. When they reached him, he was dead. The autopsy showed that he was killed by a large kidney stone which had punctured a major artery.

We have visited hot and cold water spas all over the world. The operators of these spas tell people that by drinking and bathing in these waters, various diseases will be cured. We don't believe this! Relief of pain and detoxification of body wastes from bathing in mineral water – yes! But drinking this heavy inorganic mineral water? No! It only causes serious health problems!

Our sincere and honest advice to you is:
"Don't Drink Mineralized & Fluoridated Water!"

Dolomite Limestone – Inorganic & Unhealthy

Dolomite tablets are currently sold as a magnesium and calcium supplements and are made from an inorganic limestone source. They contain the same formula that was in the feed purchased many years ago for the cattle at the Bragg family farm. The cattle absolutely refused to eat it and it was finally taken off the feed market. But now these dolomite tablets are still sold for human consumption – please avoid! **Only organic minerals can be used by the body!** You must always keep in mind that your body cannot assimilate inorganic minerals. You can only assimilate organic minerals which come from a living source (veggies, greens, sprouts, fruits, grains, nuts, herbs, etc.).

Stop Kidney Stones Cold

*Thousands upon thousands of people all over the world have kidney stones of various shapes and sizes. Sometimes these stones get so troublesome that one kidney must be removed by surgery. It is hard to believe that something as small as a kidney stone could cause such severe pain. Most people who have suffered through such an episode are highly motivated to do anything necessary to avoid another kidney stone attack. By making certain lifestyle and diet changes, kidney stone attacks can be prevented.

Kidney stones are composed of waste products – things the body doesn't use or need. Normally these wastes are eliminated through your kidneys in urine, but when there is too much waste or not enough fluid to flush it out, it all comes together to form a stone. The body is trying to push out these stones, that is what causes the excruciating pain.

You can prevent the recurrence of kidney stones by drinking eight or more 8 ounce glasses of distilled/purified water daily and eat less foods that form stones. Distilled water and healthy fluids are the most important

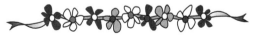

Excerpted from "No More Kidney Stones!" by John S. Rodman, M.D., R. Ernest Sosa, M.D., Cynthia Seidman, M.S., R.D. and Rory Jones

ingredients in eliminating and preventing stones. It's important to not get dehydrated and to stay away from hard and artificially softened waters and mineral waters. Salt, alcohol, colas, white sugar, white flour, inorganic calcium and animal proteins are diet "dangers" in the building stone-forming process.

Calcium is the most abundant mineral found in the kidney stones and calcium stone-formers generally have high urinary calcium. But a low-calcium diet is not recommended because of bone loss and osteoporosis. Stone-formers are urged to consume 1,000 mgs. of calcium, along with a multi-mineral supplement (see chart, page 127).

Salt (inorganic sodium) in the diet affects the way your kidneys handle calcium, causing excretion of more calcium, thus increasing your risk of forming stones. Alcohol inhibits the ability of the kidneys to excrete uric acid. It is best for your health to avoid all alcohol!!!

Kidney stones can be prevented by simply following The Bragg Healthy Lifestyle and drinking pure distilled water. Kidney stones really are "what you eat and drink!"

What is Gout?

People are sometimes disturbed when a doctor makes a diagnosis of gout to explain an aching joint, especially in their big toes. Perhaps they remember the old pictures of the British Lord with one leg wrapped up and propped on a chair in front of him, his face bearing an expression of great pain. They may also remember that he arrived at this unhappy state by living high on the hog – gorging himself on a hearty diet of animal flesh, eggs, milk and cheeses, and rich sauces and gravies made from meat . . . all washed down with chemicalized and inorganically mineralized water and maybe even some alcohol. For over 85 years, various versions of the high protein diet come and go. The purveyors of these diets rationalize that because our bodies contain a great deal of protein, we must daily eat large amounts of protein to build strong bodies (*millions of vegetarians worldwide are healthy!*). Meat protein is heavily saturated with a powerful toxic material called uric acid. Gout occurs as a result of this unbalanced disturbance in the production build-up and excretion of toxic uric acid causing health problems.

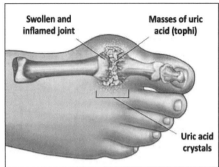

Swollen and inflamed joint

Masses of uric acid (tophi)

Uric acid crystals

After the body performs various chemical operations to break down the proteins found in all living cells, this substance – uric acid – is the final end product. A certain amount is normally found in blood, 5 or 6 milligrams per 100 milligrams of blood serum. When elevated, it increases the likelihood of gout or painful arthritis-like symptoms. How do you know if you have this problem? If you have severe, intermittent pain in a joint, most often the big toe, fingers, ankle or knee joints, your doctor may suspect joint inflammation (arthritis) known also as gouty arthritis or simply gout.

If the disease goes unchecked, the periods between attacks become shorter and the joint gradually becomes deformed. Toxic crystals formed from uric acid and inorganic minerals in hard drinking water are deposited in joints or bursa, causing destruction of surrounding tissues. These built-up tophi deposits, are also found in cartilage surrounding bone throughout the body.

The kidneys are often involved in these gouty-like disturbances. Structures within the kidneys called tubules may be blocked by the crystals deposited by uric acid and inorganic minerals. These toxic crystals are commonly reabsorbed into the body from the kidney tubules, aggravating the trouble. In fact, the most serious complication of gout is kidney damage!

Healthful Ways to Alleviate Gout

What can you do about this gouty, painful, distressing condition? It's not possible for us to offer cures, but rather to inspire you about healthy living so Mother Nature will help you clear up your health problems!

To help prevent gout and kidney stones, fast 1 day a week on 8 glasses of distilled water (cool or warm). You may add 1 to 2 teaspoons equally of organic apple cider vinegar

---

Gout is more common in males and people who drink alcohol, are obese, have diabetes, anemia and unhealthy eating habits of fast foods and soft drinks.

and raw honey to 3 of them. Drinking large amounts of pure, steam-processed distilled water often prevents the formation of kidney stones (which result from high uric acid and drinking water with inorganic minerals). Stay away from alcohol, purine foods (anchovies, gravies, kidneys, liver, meat extracts, and sardines) and salty foods. Red meats and shellfish are also no-nos for gout. Also avoid coffee, sugar, meats, fish, pork, fowl, cheese, eggs, milk and dairy products. No peas, beans and nuts, until gout is gone. The most protective foods are organic fruits and vegetables. About 60% of your diet should be raw vegetables and fruits and their fresh juices. Raw and cooked vegetables, tofu, nuts, sunflower and sesame seeds could supply protein foods (page 125). If gout conditions persist then nuts and whole grain breads should be eliminated for 6 months. Each week, faithfully undertake a 24-hour distilled water fast See web: *medicinenet.com*

Detox with an Infrared Sauna

This safe, low temperature Infrared Sauna is the best way to get rid of toxic chemicals including pesticides, heavy metals, dioxins, PCBs, plastics, inorganic minerals and hydrocarbon residues. Studies indicate sweating can off-load many of the burdens placed on the kidneys. An Infrared Sauna uses a heat energy that penetrates tissues, triggering mobilization of toxins directly into sweat. The body gets rid of stored toxins in stool, urine and sweat. (It helps if you daily take a multi-mineral supplement, especially one high in magnesium and calcium). Infrared wavelengths also lower uric acid, stimulate endorphins and kill bacteria and parasites.

We enjoyed popular saunas and steam rooms on our world travels. Gyms and Health Clubs have saunas and steam rooms. Saunas are a natural and healthy way to help restore the body to its full vitality!

Amazon Rainforest plant, Break-Stone (Chanca Piedra) promotes optimal liver, kidney and gallbladder function. It stimulates bile production and clears obstructions throughout various internal body organs. The plant is shredded and you make it as a tea – 3-4 times daily to promote cleansing and elimination of mucus, toxins, stones, and helps with gout.

Arthritis and Rheumatism

There is a bit of confusion in the use of the words rheumatism and arthritis. Nowadays, rheumatism is used loosely to mean pain and discomfort in and around the joints. In stricter usage, rheumatic conditions include not only those of bone and cartilage, but also of the tendons and tissues surrounding the bones, or their associated connective tissue. We also use the word bursitis when the inflammation is confined to the bursa, a sac containing fluid to prevent friction between a joint and tendon.

Ball and Socket

It is of sad interest to note that millions of Americans have arthritis problems, making this one of our most common physical complaints. One-tenth are disabled by arthritis to some degree. All of this indicates that arthritis, which strictly means "inflammation of the joints," is a dreaded condition! It has been estimated that there are more than 50 varieties of this disease. The kind most feared is known as rheumatoid arthritis. All ages may be *Hinge* affected. Even very young children suffer from this misery, which is often deforming.

Rheumatoid arthritis may affect different parts of the body, but the joints are the chief targets. Its onset is characterized by redness, heat and swelling, causing inflammation in one or more of the joints. When a joint is swollen and painful, it is difficult to use and therefore becomes less flexible from lack of use as well as from the misery itself. The muscles also grow smaller or atrophy without exercise. The victim may seem to *Sliding* have large and very sore joints, often with thin arms and legs.

It is within the shoulder, elbow, wrist and hand joints that inorganic minerals from salt, hard mineralized water and toxic acid crystals (from the wrong foods, etc.) may form and cripple one or more of these joints, or legs, hips, back or neck causing pain and often restricted movement.

There is no known cure for rheumatoid arthritis. We have no cures to offer you. Again, all we can offer you is The Bragg Healthy Lifestyle. Only you and the basic biological functions of your body can help you correct this unhealthy and painful condition.

Let us state emphatically that, in our opinion, the misery of arthritis is caused by ingestion of hard water saturated with inorganic minerals and toxins and an unhealthy diet. These factors combined with inactivity can form acid crystals in the moveable joints. Ill health is the result of a combination of unnatural living habits! Every effect must have a cause! There is a reason why things happen in the body. The failure to live Mother Nature's healthy lifestyle is the cause of many human miseries.

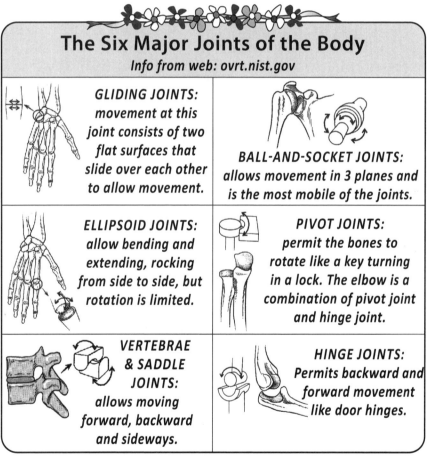

The Six Major Joints of the Body
Info from web: ovrt.nist.gov

GLIDING JOINTS: *movement at this joint consists of two flat surfaces that slide over each other to allow movement.*

BALL-AND-SOCKET JOINTS: *allows movement in 3 planes and is the most mobile of the joints.*

ELLIPSOID JOINTS: *allow bending and extending, rocking from side to side, but rotation is limited.*

PIVOT JOINTS: *permit the bones to rotate like a key turning in a lock. The elbow is a combination of pivot joint and hinge joint.*

VERTEBRAE & SADDLE JOINTS: *allows moving forward, backward and sideways.*

HINGE JOINTS: *Permits backward and forward movement like door hinges.*

Osteoporosis researchers are confirming in a variety of experiments that the more salt you eat, the more calcium you lose from your body and the more prone you become to debilitating fractures as you age.
– Tufts University Nutrition Letter – www.nutritionletter.tufts.edu

Health Hints for Aching Muscles and Joints

In order to prevent your important muscles from shriveling and becoming useless, they must be exercised. If you don't use your over 640 muscles, you lose them! Besides keeping the muscles from wasting away, gentle exercising will preserve the mobility of your joints. Even if it hurts you to exercise the affected areas, you must try to gradually work your muscles loose and flexible and your joints free of the cement-like, toxic chemical crystals. Then the toxins can be dissolved and excreted by your hard working elimination system.

Great relief from pain and swelling may be obtained through heat. Heat relieves the muscle spasms and thus improves the blood flow to both muscles and joints. Usually it is best to apply heat (via a hot bath, heating pad or heat salve – cayenne, etc.) for a little while before exercise. At the hot mineral spas in California, we saw many helpless sufferers of rheumatoid arthritis getting blessed relief from these hot mineral waters. If you can't go to a hot spring for relief, you can take a hot tub soak (massage body while soaking) adding 1 cup of Epsom salts or apple cider vinegar to water.

Natural Treatments for Pain & Inflammation

- **Omega-3 fats:** are an essential component that your body needs to reduce inflammation. Research shows that omega-3 fats and glucosamine work together to provide additional benefits for people with osteoarthritis.
- **Acupuncture/Acupressure:** are also safe and typically effective treatment methods for arthritic pain.
- **Bromelain:** This enzyme, found in pineapples, is a natural anti-inflammatory. It can be taken as a supplement, but eating fresh pineapple may be helpful.
- **Evening primrose, black currant and borage oils:** These contain the essential fatty acid gamma linolenic acid (GLA), which is useful for treating arthritic pain.

For more info see web: www.mercola.com

 Distilled water should be an important part of the treatment for arthritis, and other body ills. – Dr. Allen Banik, "Your Water & Your Health"

Check Your Mattress

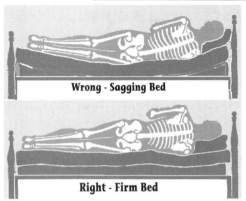

Wrong - Sagging Bed

Right - Firm Bed

Eight hours per night is the optimal amount of sleep for most adults. During sleep, you recharge the battery you ran down during the day. The right kind of mattress is important! You should sleep on a firm mattress or place a board under a soft one. This allows the muscles to stretch in natural relaxation and relieves pressure on vital organs.

Bed boards help prevent the spine from taking on curves from a soft, sagging mattress. This helps keep the spine supple and strong.

Make Sure to Stand, Walk & Sit Tall

Posture exercises to prevent a curved back and a stooped neck are excellent preventative medicine. In fact, this type of exercise should be done by everyone – even those without any sign of arthritis – to preserve the erectness of youth as long as possible. Walk, stand and sit tall! Make your muscles work to keep you stretched as tall as possible at all times! Most great men and women of history had good posture and with practice, you can too! Start now! Remember that daily good posture practice will make you more upstanding! Study the *Posture Chart* on the next page.

81

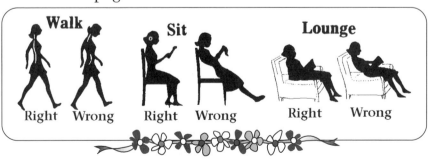

Walk Right Wrong **Sit** Right Wrong **Lounge** Right Wrong

Standing posture is important – your ears, shoulders, hips and knees should be in line with one another.

Good posture is a way of doing things with more energy, less stress and fatigue. Without good posture, you cannot really be physically fit. – hqchiro.com

WHERE DO YOU STAND?

POSTURE CHART

	PERFECT	FAIR	POOR
HEAD			
SHOULDERS			
SPINE			
HIPS			
ANKLES			
NECK			
UPPER BACK			
TRUNK			
ABDOMEN			
LOWER BACK			

82

Your posture carries you through life from your head to your feet.
This is your human vehicle and you are truly a miracle! Cherish, respect
and always protect it by living The Bragg Healthy Lifestyle. – Patricia Bragg

Good posture helps prevent backaches and related problems.

Remember – Your posture can make or break your health!

POSTURE SILHOUETTES: Which one are you?

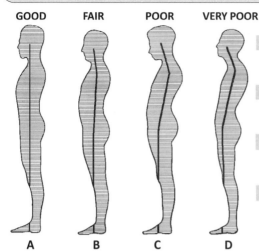

GOOD   FAIR   POOR   VERY POOR

A GOOD: Head, trunk and thigh in a straight line; chest high and forward; abdomen flat; back curves normally.

B FAIR: Head too forward; abdomen too prominent; exaggerated curve in upper back; slightly hollow lower back.

C POOR: Relaxed posture; head too forward; abdomen relaxed; shoulder blades prominent; hollow lower back.

D VERY POOR: Head too far forward; very exaggerated curve in upper back; abdomen relaxed; chest flat-sloping;

A   B   C   D

Doomed to Human Scrap Pile

Most big corporations are less likely to hire someone who is 50 years of age. They know from actual experience that there is considerable brain deterioration and brain slow down in the majority of unhealthy people over 50.

It all boils down to simple physics (basic physiological facts). You have small blood vessels leading to your brain. The way the average person avoids exercise, eats junk and drinks hard water invites degenerative changes in these blood vessels throughout the body and especially in the brain. The longer the average person lives in this manner, the more body degeneration takes place!

Many senior citizens will admit that their mental faculties seem to be slipping. They will tell you how poor their memory has become and how they cannot always recall names and events. A brain turning to stone does not have the capacity to be wide awake and sharp! As this condition gets worse, we call it senility. In time, the brain solidifies to a point where it remembers nothing. This is called living in deep senility or dementia. Or is it a living death?

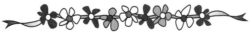

Every man is the builder of a temple called his body . . . we are all sculptors and painters and our material is our own flesh and blood and bones.
– Henry David Thoreau, American author, poet, philosopher

How the Brain Functions

Did you ever stop to consider what makes you think? Inside the protective covering of the bony skull is a mass of what we call "gray matter." Gray matter is tissue composed of millions of nerve cells "woven" together – enabling what we see, hear, taste and touch to give us an awareness of our status on this beautiful earth.

Using our gray matter, we also think, know, remember, judge and believe. It was named gray matter because it is largely pinkish-gray in color. The brain also has a white part. Our behavior and emotions are controlled by this mass of tissue. We now know that the secretions of the endocrine glands also affect the mainstream of these communications, which in turn alters brain cells.

This miracle computer, the brain, is an incredibly complex electrochemical organ, as individual to each of us as are our fingerprints! It's the miracle of life which gives us love, joy and sorrow, philosophy and politics, understanding and reasoning power, will power and the ability to have many feelings. Philosophers have called it "man's unconquerable mind." As we see what has been developed by it from one century to another, we can almost call the adjective "unconquerable" a factual one.

As the average person's brain slowly turns to stone, much of their birthright of keen awareness becomes lost. Eyesight starts to go as cataracts develop (a stony film formation over the eyes). Hearing becomes impaired because the arteries leading to the ears become corroded with inorganic mineral encrustations. These are all diseases of degeneration, which most people blame on the passing years, not on how badly they have lived.

This amazing gray matter we call the brain must have oxygenated blood or it degenerates! All living cells of the body must have oxygen in large quantities to survive. Senility is caused by the oxygen starvation of the brain.

There's nothing wrong with looking as youthful as you can regardless of your chronological age. When you're healthy, you look and feel young and there is nothing wrong with that! – Dr. Howard Murad

Cross Section of Human Brain

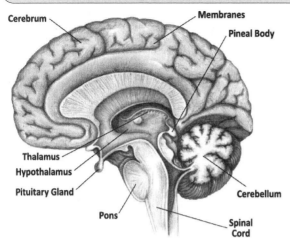

Cerebrum
Membranes
Pineal Body
Thalamus
Hypothalamus
Pituitary Gland
Pons
Cerebellum
Spinal Cord

Adult Brain

The adult brain, the human computer, weighs about 3 lbs., but it powerfully directs all of your thoughts, feelings and actions.

To possess an ageless and unconquerable mind, we must constantly provide it with a free flow of life-giving, oxygen-rich, red blood. That is the reason the supply pipes leading to the brain must not be blocked by encrusted inorganic minerals. If you wish to maintain or regain a strong brain, use only steam-produced distilled water and fresh fruit and vegetable juices as your drinks. Please keep far away from city, well and tap waters, alcohol, tea, coffee, cola, diet and soda drinks.

85

The Brain Needs High Quality Nutrition

The brain must be adequately nourished in order to function properly. No other part of the body fails more quickly from lack of good nutrition. Upon what does this marvelous structure feed? It needs foods rich in enzymes. Organic raw fruits and vegetables and their fresh juices provide excellent nourishment. Soy beans, which are exceptionally rich in lecithin, should be eaten several times weekly. Lecithin in powdered, liquid, capsule, tablet or granulated form can also be purchased at your health food store. Raw, unsalted sunflower, sesame and pumpkin seeds are all healthful brain foods.

The brain is the most complex organ in the body. It is the organ that allows us to think, feel, move and dream. – BrainHealthAndPuzzles.com

Keep it youthful – Cross-Train your brain with family and friends, exchange ideas and learn new challenges, games, sports, dances, etc.

Brain Control Areas

FRONTAL LOBE

PARIETAL LOBE

INTELLECT
WRITING
MOTOR
SPEECH
TOE
LEG
ARM
FACE
TONGUE
SENSATION

HEARING
TASTE
SMELL
AUDITORY SPEECH
VISUAL SPEECH
SIGHT

OCCIPITAL LOBE

PONS
CEREBELLUM
OBLONGATA

TEMPORAL LOBE

Everything you do – including seeing, hearing, speaking, breathing & moving – is controlled by a part of your brain as shown here.

Organic Minerals are Essential to Life

86

The brain needs phosphorus. Organic phosphorus is found in beans of all kinds including: pinto, garbanzo and dried lima beans and lentils. Other phosphorus rich sources are: 100% whole grains, brown rice, almonds, peanuts and walnuts. Lean meats, egg yolks and natural, unprocessed cheeses also contain organic phosphorus.

All of the organic minerals are needed to keep the body strong, youthful and healthy. They are essential factors in digestion and assimilation, constituting important ingredients of the digestive juices and regulating the osmotic exchange between lymph and blood cells. In short, organic minerals are indispensable to the proper physiological functioning of all the systems of the body.

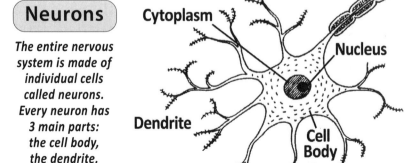

Neurons

The entire nervous system is made of individual cells called neurons. Every neuron has 3 main parts: the cell body, the dendrite, and the axon

Axon

Cytoplasm

Nucleus

Dendrite

Cell Body

Organic Minerals Make the Man!

It's estimated that an average man weighing about 150 pounds is composed of the following:

90 lbs. oxygen
36 lbs. carbon
14 lbs. hydrogen
3 lbs. 8 oz. nitrogen
3 lbs. 12 oz. calcium
1 lb. 4 oz. phosphorus
3½ oz. sulphur
3 oz. potassium
2½ oz. sodium
1½ oz. magnesium
¼ oz. silicon
1/16 oz. iron

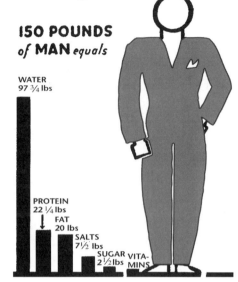

150 POUNDS *of* **MAN** *equals*

WATER
97 ¾ lbs

PROTEIN
22 ¼ lbs
FAT
20 lbs
SALTS
7½ lbs
SUGAR VITA-
2½ lbs MINS

trace amounts of these other important elements include: manganese, zinc, neon, iodine, copper, lithium, cobalt, helium.

The Body is Composed of Organic Minerals

Remember that these are **ALL ORGANIC** – not inorganic – chemicals and minerals. There is a sharp line of demarcation between the two! Although the chemical analysis is the same whether found in air, earth, plant or animal – it is only through the life processes of the plant whereby the constituents of air and soil become vitalized and useful to the human body. It is this property of vitality alone which distinguishes, for example, the atom of iron in the red corpuscles of the blood from that of inorganic iron or preparations made from inorganic iron. You could suck on an iron nail for years and never extract any organic iron for building your blood. When you eat blackberries, you are getting organic iron that can be used by the blood. The arrangement of atoms that form a molecule of the iron nail is the same as that of the organic iron in the blackberry. Only by the great natural miracle force of photosynthesis does the living plant convert the inert inorganic minerals into the organic minerals which we can use for keeping ourselves alive and healthy!

Formula for Creating a Human Being

According to Bernard Alwyne Howard – in his book *The Proper Study of Mankind* – the human body contains:

- Enough water to fill a 10 gallon barrel.
- Enough fat to make 7 bars of soap.
- Enough carbon for 9,000 lead pencils.
- Enough phosphorus for 2,200 match-heads.
- Just enough iron for 1 medium-size nail.
- Enough calcium (lime) to whitewash a chicken coop.
- And microscopic amounts of such trace elements as cobalt, iodine, zinc, copper, molybdenum, titanium, beryllium, etc.

Take these ingredients; combine them in the right proportions and in the right way; and the result, apparently, is the creation of a man, claims Howard.

Bragg Motto – Live Foods Make Live People

Sometimes the minerals of the body are referred to as "mineral salts." This misleading terminology has given the public the wrong idea that this term "salt" refers to common table salt, or inorganic sodium chloride. Most people mistakenly consider added salt an indispensable adjunct to almost all foods and part of a healthy diet. The fact cannot be over-emphasized that there is a vital change going on in all the minerals as they are absorbed into the structure of the plant. On the other hand, chemical analysis or separation of the minerals means destruction of the living tissues. But of course, the chemist will find in the minerals of the "ash" those same properties that are present in the minerals of the soil. But that subtle, imponderable force – vital electricity (the life force of plants) – has escaped him. It cannot be isolated by the laboratory processes of condensation or the extraction. We must learn to recognize the body's mineral elements as being "organic" components – internal parts of the living body and subject to the same vital changes, life and death, that affect the organism.

Nature, the ocean, and life are divine mysteries. – see wyland.com (page 169)

The organic calcium in the skeleton, the organic iron contained in the red corpuscles and the organic sodium and potassium found in the blood serum are biologically organized. They have a certain duration of life during which they have vital functions to perform. Sooner or later these molecules will lose their electromagnetic tension, according to the degree of their physiological activity. In other words, they have served their purpose and must be supplanted by fresh organic minerals. **That is the reason that 60% –70% of your diet should be fresh, organic raw fruits and vegetables.** These are the great suppliers of the imponderable life force – vital electricity.

The Alkaline or Base-Forming Minerals

The alkaline minerals – which are so important in the performance of the physiological functions of the body are iron, sodium, calcium, magnesium, potassium and manganese. These are the eliminators of toxic waste poisons, the real immunizers of the body. They are essential to the formation of the digestive juices and the secretions of the ductless glands. (These hormones regulate nearly all the vital processes of the body.)

Iron is necessary for the formation of the red blood corpuscles and acts as the oxygen carrier of the system. Elimination of carbon dioxide depends largely upon organic sodium, which is the chief constituent of the blood and lymph. Calcium, combined with magnesium, phosphorus and silicon, makes up more than half of the bony structure of the body and imparts strength to all tissues. It also serves as a neutralizer and eliminator of toxic acids. Remember, whenever we refer to minerals in the body, we are speaking of the organic minerals.

There are no more important ingredients of a properly constituted diet than organic fruits and vegetables, for they naturally contain vitamins and minerals of every class, recognized and unrecognized. – Sir Robert McCarrison

---

It's a mistake to think that the more a man eats, the stronger he will become.

Vegetarians have denser, better formed bones and stronger immune systems! – Linda Page, Ph.D., Author "Healthy Healing" • HealthyHealing.com

---

Nature never deceives us; it is always we who deceive ourselves. – Rousseau

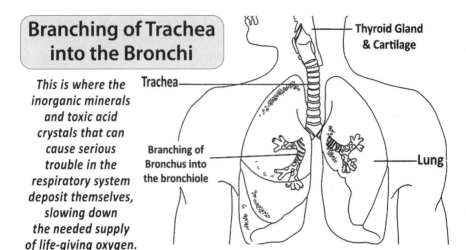

Branching of Trachea into the Bronchi

Thyroid Gland & Cartilage

Trachea

This is where the inorganic minerals and toxic acid crystals that can cause serious trouble in the respiratory system deposit themselves, slowing down the needed supply of life-giving oxygen.

Branching of Bronchus into the bronchiole

Lung

Water – Curse of Millions of Aching Backs

By the time they reach 40, millions of Americans are plagued by lower back pains. When they bend over it is absolute agony! Their whole lower spine is becoming fossilized and cemented with inorganic calcification.

Many people by 40 have worn out much of the cartilage that acts as a cushion to the spinal bones. This is a painful condition that only gets progressively worse on a constant diet of chemicalized and mineralized water. Plus, most suffer from extreme dehydration that, combined with their unhealthy acid crystal-forming diet, adds to their overall joint and health problems.

Inorganic Mineral Water, Spring, Well, River, Lake & Faucet Water You Drink Can Turn You to Stone!

When Dad was a small boy, his father took him and the other children of the family to Washington, D.C., to see the P.T. Barnum Circus.

To a young boy this was a great event! After seeing the big circus show in the big tent, they all visited the "Side Show" tent where all the unusual, so-called circus "freaks" were exhibited. There were fat men and women – some weighing as much as 600 pounds – dwarfs, giants, the bearded lady, the monkey man and others.

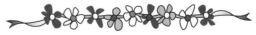

Happiness is not being pained in body or troubled in mind. – Thomas Jefferson

But the one that most fascinated my dad was the lady who had turned to stone. There was a woman on a bed who was so full of arthritis and acid crystals that she had no feeling left in her petrified body. She lay helpless and rigid. She could move only her eyes. This lady suffered from complete ankylosis – meaning that no joint in her entire body could make a simple movement. All the nerve tissue in her body was paralyzed and dead – they could actually drive nails into her body! The man who explained these "freaks" said that this lady was born in Hot Springs, Arkansas, which explained it, as my father later discovered.

Stone Lady Mystery Solved

The lady who had turned to stone was a complete mystery to my father as a child. But not today! The water in Hot Springs is some of the hardest water in the United States. We have seen chemical analyses of it and the concentrations of calcium carbonate, potassium carbonate and magnesium carbonate are very, very high. That poor lady in the side show was a victim of this inorganic water. Her vital organs were not strong enough to flush those inorganic minerals out of her body, so they deposited themselves in her joints. This was an unusual and extreme case, of course. But we've seen many, many cases of arthritics who were complete cripples, absolutely helpless. There are more than 91 million people young and old living in the United States today who suffer from arthritis to some degree.

91

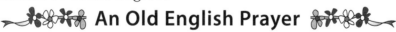 **An Old English Prayer**

Give us Lord, a bit of sun,
A bit of work and a bit of fun.

Give us in all the struggle and sputter,
Our daily whole grain bread and food.

Give us health, our keep to make
And a bit to spare for others' sake.

Give us too, a bit of song,
And a tale and a book, to help us along.

Give us Lord, a chance to be
Our goodly best for ourselves and others,
Until men learn to live as brothers.

Do-It-Yourself Calcification Test

Take this simple test to discover just how calcified your various body joints have become:

Stand erect, hands hanging loosely at your sides. Now lower your head to your chest and start a slow rolling movement, around and around. Many people can feel the inorganic calcification grating as they roll their head. This shows that there has been a definite infiltration of insoluble minerals and toxic acid crystals into the axis of the important atlas, the bone at the top of the spine upon which your skull rests.

Also test the moveable joints of your body: Do you have stiffness? How limber is your spine? Can you raise your hands over your head and bend forward with your knees locked to touch the floor with your fingertips? Are you limber enough to place the palms of your hands on the floor as you keep your knees stiff?

Stand with your back to a wall. Move forward about 2 feet, then bend backward and "walk" down the wall with your hands. How far can you go?

How high can you kick? Do you have cracking in your knees when you do a leg squat? How flexible are your bare feet? Do you walk with a spring in your step? Do you have a feeling of suppleness and flexibility in your body? Do you walk and dance with grace, or do you walk on calcified encrustations that cause you misery and pain? Is your body flexible and pain-free?

Don't say your stiffness is due to your age! That is so much rubbish! You can keep your body youthful and flexible with proper care, living The Bragg Healthy Lifestyle!

It is never too late to begin getting into shape, but it does take daily exercise and strong perseverance.
– Thomas K. Cureton, pioneer physical fitness researcher

Perfection consists not in doing extraordinary things, but in doing ordinary things extraordinarily well. Neglect nothing; the most trivial action may be performed with joy.
– Jacqueline Marie Angélique Arnauld

The unexamined life is not worth living. It is time to re-evaluate your past as a guide to your future. – Socrates

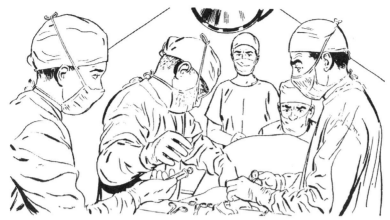

There are over 6,000 hospitals in the U.S. where surgery goes on around the clock. Many people undergo orthopedic surgery to have joint replacements and painful bone spurs removed, as well as bladder stones, kidney stones and gallstones. Will you be next? Web: HospitalLink.com

Bone Spurs and Moveable Joint Calcification

Every day large numbers of people go into surgery to have joint replacements or to have painful, crippling bone spurs removed or to have calcified deposits removed from their moveable joints. These bone spurs and calcified formations are insoluble deposits that get into the tissues after consumption of water loaded with inorganic minerals, salt and uric acid, plus deposited toxic acid crystals from an incorrect diet high in acid. Meat, refined flour products, white bread, coffee, sodas and sugary desserts are all high in acid content. This is the unhealthy dead-food diet that most people eat. This diet, combined with hard water, is why there are many joint troubles resulting from acid deposits that create bone spurs and painful crystallized joints, etc.

93

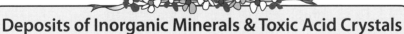

Deposits of Inorganic Minerals & Toxic Acid Crystals

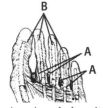

*Inorganic mineral deposits that deposit themselves between the bones of the toes (**A** and **B**).*

A. Deposited under tendons

B. Under the Achilles tendon

C. Under the heel

D. Under the middle foot

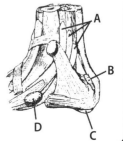

Inorganic Deposits Cause Bad Posture

Inorganic minerals and toxic acid crystals are a major cause of poor posture. This can bring on all sorts of bad disturbances by throwing the vital organs out of place, unduly straining some muscles, while weakening others, impairing circulation, breathing and elimination. Just stand on any busy city corner and watch the people of all ages shuffle by you. What a miserable sight most of them present – people whose feet are so loaded with inorganic calcification and pain that they simply lift their feet up and put them down! The spring's absolutely gone from their step.

Many people walk like ducks with their toes pointing outward. Others walk stooped and are bent out of shape. Some walk stiff with no knee action. You see many whose steps are unsteady because their joints are so cemented and others who are so out of balance that they sway from side to side as they hobble along. Their heads are carried too far forward, throwing their bodies off balance. Watch them as they try to sit down. They simply plop into the chair, giving their lower back and hips a shock.

94

Calcified Toenails and Fingernails

Inorganic minerals, salt and toxic acid crystals can deform the toes and fingernails. We've both seen toes and fingers that were made into monstrosities by calcified joints and nails. Thick toenails that are hard as cement that usually no pair of scissors or clippers can cut them and they have to be filed down with a rugged file. They can often deform the feet, making walking extremely painful, while presenting an unattractive appearance. Read Bragg Back & Foot Book (see page 196) for more information on the feet.

In most cases, toxic acid crystals can be removed by the person themselves with a careful hygienic foot plan. This includes a health hygiene with foot therapy, water treatment, massage, reflexology, exercise, natural nutrition and some fasting. – Excerpt from Bragg Back & Foot Book

---

Healthy body, bones & feet come from healthy foods, habits & lifestyle.
– Patricia Bragg, Health Crusader

Cold Feet and Cold Hands

Many people of all ages suffer from poor circulation, in many cases due to or aggravated by inorganic mineral encrustations in the arteries, veins and capillaries that constitute the blood circulatory system.

We have frequently shaken hands with people whose hands were ice cold even on the warmest days. Many people also suffer from extremely cold feet, especially in cold weather. By age 60, many people have patches of small blue, broken and expanded veins around their feet, ankles, and legs, giving an appearance of bruising, blackness or dirtiness, even just after a bath.

Poor circulation is first and most critically noticeable in the hands and feet because the blood has farther to go from the heart to reach these extremities. When the pipes of the body become clogged and obstructed, the blood has difficulty in getting through. Instead of coursing through the capillaries of the hands and feet in a warm, healthy stream, it trickles through – barely able to bring nourishment, much less any warmth.

The entire body, of course, is affected when the pipes of the circulatory system are clogged. People with poor circulation find it difficult to keep warm in cold or even cool weather. Their overheated homes become like a hothouse living arena. They must bundle up in sweaters, coats and bulky clothing when they go outside.

Every sick person usually has a sluggish circulatory system that is operating on a very low level – chiefly due to plugged-up pipes. Remember that the main source of these encrustations is drinking water saturated with inorganic minerals. Those who drink distilled water and the juices of fruits and vegetables are helping to keep their circulatory systems clean and more healthy.

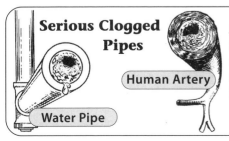

Serious Clogged Pipes

Human Artery

Water Pipe

An artery with heavy internal deposits can be compared to scale that forms on the inside of a water pipe. An artery clogged like this results in an increase in blood pressure and may cause a heart attack or stroke.

Exercises for Healthy Feet

> **Do these simple exercises daily to help keep feet in good healthy condition and improve circulation:**

1. Toe exercise: raise weight of the body up on toes.
2. Grasp with your toes, pick up a pencil, etc.
3. Sitting in chair with legs outstretched, curl toes up and then stretch toes down and under.
4. In same position as #3, rotate feet clockwise several times. Then repeat, rotating feet counterclockwise.
5. Sit on floor with soles of feet together; pull the heels and toes alternately apart.
6. Stand with your feet parallel, 5 to 6 inches apart; bend the knees and turn them outward while keeping the feet flat on the floor and bend down slightly.
7. Walk barefooted on soft grass or sand anytime the opportunity arises. Your feet love contact with the earth, plus the exercise and the increase in circulation all help to build happy, healthy feet.
8. As soon as you come into the house you should remove your shoes – remember, barefooted is best!
9. Give yourself or your partner first a vinegar foot soak (2 Tbsps ACV in hot water) then a foot massage while watching TV or listening to music – rotate, work, kneed and apply pressure to soles and toes for healing delights.

96

Not only do foot soaks and massages help tired and aching feet, but elevating the feet by putting them up on wall, back of couch or by holding them in air for ten minutes helps reduce congestion and varicose veins. Resting the feet is as important as resting the body!

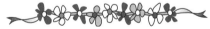

For more foot and vinegar treatments read the Bragg Book
"Apple Cider Vinegar – Miracle Health System." – See back pages

---

The healing power of massage reduces stress, back and foot pain, and helps fight depression, fatigue, anxiety and helps save lives. – Patricia Bragg

---

A wise man should consider that health is the greatest of human blessings!
– Hippocrates, Father of Medicine, 400 B.C.

Disfiguring Broken Capillaries

Among the many manifestations of inorganic calcification are broken facial capillaries. Study people's faces. Look closely at the cheek, around the nose and on the chin, where you will often see the smallest blood vessels, slender as hairs, showing near the surface of the skin. When tiny capillaries become encrusted with inorganic minerals, even alcohol, they expand and often rupture, making purplish or reddish blotches. Blocked by inorganic minerals and no longer able to handle the circulation of the blood, except perhaps to a small degree, these broken capillaries not only give the face an unhealthy appearance, but are often quite painful.

Head Noises and Ringing in Ears

Many humans are plagued by head noises, ringing and pounding in the ears. Every waking hour is torture as these head noises wear down their nerve energy. Even in sleep, they have bad dreams about these noises. These head noises may torment them 24 hours a day.

The blood vessels – arteries, veins and capillaries – in the delicate canals of the ears have become hardened and obstructed by inorganic mineral encrustations from hard water, as well as uric acid and deposits of toxic acid crystals from unbalanced diets. This condition produces the head noises – buzzing sounds, ringing and pounding in the ears.

In time, the blood vessels of the ears become so clogged that the person gradually goes deaf. Millions of people start going deaf every year for this reason alone! For a time, they can get some relief from a hearing aid, but many will eventually lose their hearing completely.

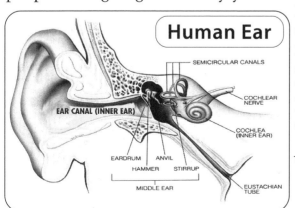

Human Ear

SEMICIRCULAR CANALS

COCHLEAR NERVE

EAR CANAL (INNER EAR)

COCHLEA (INNER EAR)

EARDRUM   ANVIL

HAMMER   STIRRUP

MIDDLE EAR

EUSTACHIAN TUBE

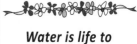

Water is life to all living things.

Inorganic Minerals and Toxins Affect Eyes

Inorganic minerals, toxic poisons and uric acid also have a degenerative effect upon the eyes. Your eyes are among your most important physical possessions. They are often described as the mirror of the soul, the mind and the thoughts. It is true that your eyes often reveal your innermost feelings. Their lustre changes because of psychological influences – such as fear, love, hatred – and because of physical malfunctions. Without your eyes, you would live in total darkness. Many people do!

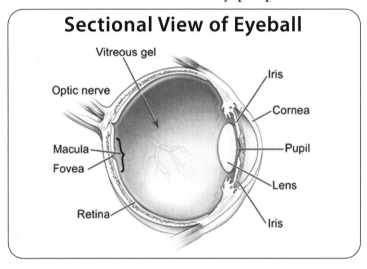

Sectional View of Eyeball

Vitreous gel

Optic nerve

Iris

Cornea

Macula

Fovea

Pupil

Lens

Retina

Iris

Now let us examine this miracle mechanism – the eye. The eyeball is an almost spherical body with a mirror at the back portion, the retina. The body of the eye is made up of a transparent jelly-like substance. From the back of the eye runs the optic sensory nerve. This is a head nerve, a major part of the central nervous system.

In the front of the eye there is a crystalline biconvex lens, which is more convex behind the cornea. The white portion of the eye is a fibrous material surrounding the central, colored part – varying in shades of brown, blue, hazel or gray – known as the iris. The iris serves as a photosensitive diaphragm, controlling the amount of light which enters the pupil, the black spot in the center of the eye. When the outside light is bright, the muscles of the iris contract the pupil to a small dot. When the outside light grows dimmer, the pupil expands proportionally to admit more light.

Natural Foods Help Protect Your Eyes

The eye is a delicate mechanism. All the blood vessels which bring needed nourishment and oxygen to the eye are very tiny capillaries. Year after year, most people drink chemicalized and inorganically mineralized water and absorb toxic uric acids from their foods. Just as in limestone caverns the stalactites and stalagmites are formed drop by drop, so the blood deposits inorganic minerals and toxic acids slowly into the eyes' tiny blood capillaries. Encrustations are slowly formed in these delicate capillaries. Glasses are prescribed, after time stronger glasses. Then vision starts to fail and, in some cases, a person is left in total darkness.

Many people panic when they start losing their precious vision. They try treatments of all kinds, even operations, but their sight gradually fades. Remember avoid these vicious enemies of healthy eyes: unhealthy foods, fluoride, chlorine, inorganic mineral water, toxic poisons from acid-forming foods and uric acid from a diet too heavy in animal proteins.

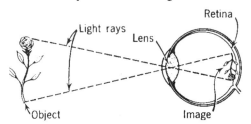

The Human Eye is like a camera. Light rays enter the eye, cross in the lens and focus on the retina.

Build Clean, Healthy Blood For Health

The blood holds the key to our health, vitality and our youthfulness – and our very life! **Keep the blood free from inorganic minerals and toxic acids!**

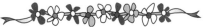

Lutein helps keep eyes healthier and is concentrated mostly in the retina and lens. Lutein is found naturally in fruits and leafy green vegetables. Vitamin A, C, and Ds are important in preventing cataracts and Macular Degeneration. Vitamin D3 found in sunshine and (3,000 IU's) are desirable for eye, bone, heart and skin health. Vitamin A is found in sweet potatoes, carrots, mangoes and dried apricots. Vitamin C is high in oranges and strawberries.

Nothing can bring you peace but yourself. – Ralph Waldo Emerson

DIAGRAM OF THE CIRCULATORY SYSTEM

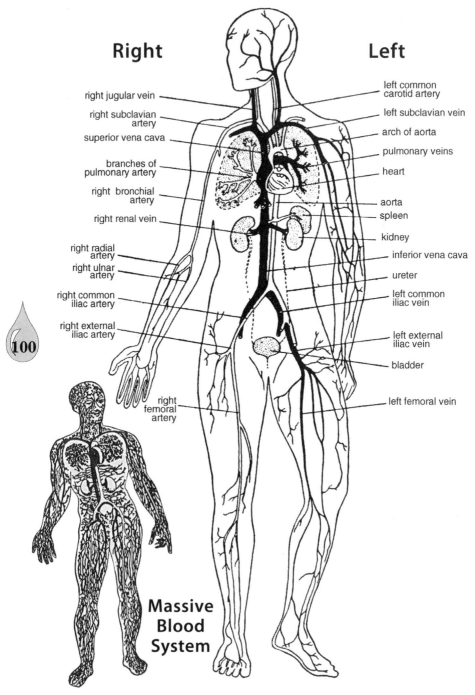

Right

Left

right jugular vein

right subclavian artery

superior vena cava

branches of pulmonary artery

right bronchial artery

right renal vein

right radial artery

right ulnar artery

right common iliac artery

right external iliac artery

100

right femoral artery

left common carotid artery

left subclavian vein

arch of aorta

pulmonary veins

heart

aorta

spleen

kidney

inferior vena cava

ureter

left common iliac vein

left external iliac vein

bladder

left femoral vein

Massive Blood System

For the sake of clarity most blood vessels are not shown on the larger art. We show only some of the arteries and veins. The smaller art shows the entire body blood system.

Every 90 days we build a brand new bloodstream. We can live and regain health using a reversal program being careful of the kind of water we drink and the kind of foods we eat! Starting today discard materials which create an unhealthy bloodstream and start building one with natural foods that promote a painless, tireless and ageless body! It's all up to you!

Using the knowledge offered in this book, you can start becoming more youthful as you live longer. You must be the absolute master of what goes into your body in the way of food and drink. Flesh is dumb! Your body will accept almost all foods. That is the reason **you must read this book several times and start living The Bragg Healthy Lifestyle for building clean, healthy blood!**

Of course, we all know what blood looks like . . . a somewhat thickish red fluid that we see whenever the skin is even slightly broken. These tiny oozings of blood come from very tiny blood vessels which supply the skin all over the body. Blood, your 'River of Life', is the fluid which carries oxygen and nutrition to all the cells of the body and tries to remove any poisonous substances. The trouble is that the average person keeps pouring inorganic minerals and toxic poisons into the body so fast that the blood finds it impossible to purify itself, much less the body. Nothing could be more important than this "life blood" of ours. If we do not get enough oxygen and nutrition and if toxic materials are not removed regularly, they will stockpile and we will die.

And that, we are sorry to say, is why many die long before their time. People do not take the time to learn how to get more oxygen into the body; they do not take time or interest in good nutrition. Death comes from accumulated toxins that actually poison and clog up the bloodstream, brain, organs and nervous system. The heavy concentrations of inorganic minerals, salt, fat and toxic poisons which are a burden to the body are the vicious killers! Years are not your enemies! It's what you put into your body that does the terrible damage to your health and erodes your future longevity!

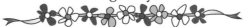

Pure distilled water is truly God's greatest gift to us – it's the vital natural chemistry of life, and a source of health. – Paul C. Bragg, N.D., Ph.D.

Exercise and Eat for Total Health

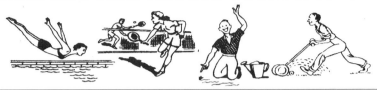

Enjoy Bragg Healthy Lifestyle
For a Lifetime of Super Health

In a broad sense, The Bragg Healthy Lifestyle for the Total Person is a combination of physical, mental, emotional, social and spiritual components. The ability of the individual to function effectively in his environment depends on how smoothly these components function as a whole. Of all the qualities that comprise an integrated personality, a totally healthy, fit body is one of the most desirable . . . so start today to achieve your health goals!

A person may be said to be totally physically fit if he functions as a total personality with efficiency and without pain or discomfort of any kind. This is to have a painless, tireless, ageless body. One possessing sufficient muscular strength and endurance to maintain a healthy posture and successfully carry on the duties imposed by life and the environment. To be able to handle emergencies and have enough energy for recreation and social obligations after the "work day" has ended. It is to meet the requirements of his environment through possessing the resilience to recover rapidly from fatigue, tension, stress and strain of daily living without the aid of stimulants, drugs or alcohol. To be able to enjoy natural recharging sleep at night and awaken fit and alert in the morning for the challenges of the new fresh day ahead.

Keeping the body totally healthy and fit is not a job for the uninformed or the careless person. It requires an understanding of the body and of a healthy lifestyle and then following it for a long, happy lifetime of health! The result of "The Bragg Healthy Lifestyle" is to wake up the possibilities within you, rejuvenate your body, mind and soul to total balanced health. It's within your reach, so don't procrastinate, start today! Our hearts and prayers go out to touch you with nourishing, caring love for your total health and life!

Patricia Bragg and *Paul C. Bragg*

Chapter 7

Organic Minerals

Iron, the Oxygen Carrier of the Blood

Organic iron is indispensable to the formation of chlorophyll and hemoglobin. Because of its great affinity for oxygen, iron plays an important part in the organic world. It has a very close relationship to the fundamental processes of biological transformation of matter known as metabolism.

The plant or tree takes the inorganic iron from the soil. It carries the iron to the leaves where it takes part in the formation of chlorophyll granules (*this green matter is the blood of plants*). The amounts of organic iron and chlorophyll vary in different parts of the plant. For instance, the green outer leaves of cabbage contain four times as much iron as the inner leaves.

How Plants Do Their Miracle Work

In order to carry out their miracle life processes, every organism is equipped with structures enabling it to use the materials in its environment to satisfy and meet its needs. Animals, with their power of locomotion, are able to hunt for food. Plants, lacking this ability, must have some way of procuring food from their immediate surroundings. In the highly developed plants, the structures particularly fitted for this purpose are the root, stem and leaf. The root, besides anchoring the plant in the soil, takes in water and minerals. The leaf, being rich in chlorophyll (*it's blood*), carries out the process of photosynthesis by uniting the water absorbed by the roots with carbon dioxide gathered from the atmosphere. This miracle process produces simple sugar, an organic rich food for the plant.

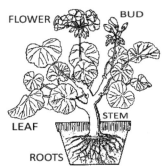

Everything in excess is opposed by nature.
– Hippocrates, Father of Medicine

The stem is an intermediate structure which conducts the water from the root to the leaf. It holds the leaf in the best position for it to receive maximum sunlight. The stem also carries the newly manufactured sugar from the leaf to various places in the plant where it can be stored for future use. Plants, vegetables, trees and flowers are all miracles!

Iron Serves Four Distinct Purposes In Plants, Animals and Man

1. Iron produces the chlorophyll (blood) of the plant, principally contained in the green leaves, and the hemoglobin of the red corpuscles in man.

2. Iron enables the plant to take carbon dioxide and nitrogen from the air and to synthesize them into organic matter using chlorophyll and sunlight.

3. Iron assists in the processes of respiration in man and animals. It is the hemoglobin that carries the oxygen to all parts of the body, reaching every cell through the capillaries. Here the carbon of the ingested food, stored in the cells of the tissues, is oxidized and changed into carbonic acid. This in turn is combined with the alkaline elements of the blood and eliminated through the constant working lungs.

4. Iron generates a magnetic blood current and an electromagnetic induction current in the nerve spirals which pass through the walls of the arteries and veins, helping to build and nourish the tissues.

The total amount of iron in the human body is comparatively small. Under normal conditions, it does not exceed 75 grains. Of this quantity, about 50 grains are contained in the blood, with the remainder being distributed throughout the marrow of the bones, in the liver and principally in the spleen. Iron is the most active mineral in the system, and therefore needs to be renewed more frequently than the more stable elements of calcium and potassium in the bones and tissues.

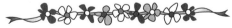

 The treatment of diseases should go to the root cause. Most often it is found in severe dehydration from lack of sufficient water and living an unhealthy lifestyle!

The quantity of blood in a 160 pound normal adult man is about 12 pounds (7.5% of body weight) and contains approximately 50 grains of iron. With every pulse beat, nearly 6 ounces of blood are forced from the heart into our major artery, the aorta. Every 30 seconds, that blood passes from the heart into the lungs. Then the blood travels from the lungs into the arteries and capillaries throughout the body. Consequently, these 50 grains of iron pass through the heart and lungs 120 times per hour, or 2,880 times per day. Within 24 hours under normal conditions, the 50 grains of iron have to perform the same function as 2,880 x 50 grains, or more than 20 pounds! For that reason alone, a daily supply of organic iron in our food is essential to the body.

Organic Vegetables and Fruits are Good, Heathy Sources of Iron

The best organic iron sources are organically grown green leafy vegetables, raw spinach (raw is best since cooked spinach has some oxalic acid), parsley, watercress, sprouts, raw squash, Swiss chard, dandelion and mustard greens, green cabbage, leeks, sorrel, Bibb lettuce, green lettuce, the skins of unwaxed cucumbers, avocado, horseradish, beet greens, artichokes, asparagus, carrots, tomatoes, beets, corn, black radish, pumpkin and corn.

105

Many fresh organically grown fruits and their juices have a high content of organic iron. Leading the list are blackberries, raspberries, blueberries, gooseberries, and grapes, cherries, oranges, peaches, strawberries and pears. Natural sun-dried fruits are high in iron – with apricots being highest (our favorite), followed by black figs, prunes, peaches, dates and raisins. Many other foods have a high content of iron: blackstrap and Barbados molasses, raw wheat germ, soy beans, raw and unsalted sesame, pumpkin, sunflower seeds and nutritional yeast, whole barley, dried beans of all kinds (pinto, kidney, lima, lentils, garbanzos), raw and unsalted nuts, natural brown rice, dried peas, rice bran, wheat bran, rye, whole grain cereals and millet. All these foods will have a higher content of iron if grown organically with no chemical

---

Only I can change my life. No one else can do it for me. – Carol Burnett

fertilizers and absolutely no poisonous sprays. Let us again impress upon you that your body needs **organic** iron – not the iron that comes from inorganic sources.

Can our bodies get iron from water? You often hear about a certain well or spring containing large amounts of iron. Some water does contain inorganic iron. But your body cannot use this inorganic iron – in fact, this iron is dangerous to your body! It can cause all kinds of stones to form in your vital organs, cement your joints and could turn your blood vessels to stone. Again we caution you to: **Stay away from inorganic minerals!**

Every Mineral Matters

The body contains 19 essential mineral elements, all of which must be derived from live foods. Calcium, phosphorus and magnesium are vital for the growth and maintenance of bone; potassium and organic sodium give your body fluids for composition and stability. Phosphorus, calcium and sulphur are the essential constituents of the body cells from which all organs and tissues are composed.

Magnesium, iron and phosphorus are important to help with the release of energy from your food. Iodine (*seaweed and kelp*) is important to the thyroid gland, which controls growth and the rate at which energy is used. Copper and iron minerals are needed in forming the red blood cells.

Other minerals like sulphur and cobalt are used in the synthesis of some vitamins by the body. Zinc is an essential part of the insulin

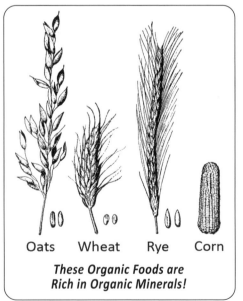

Oats   Wheat   Rye   Corn

These Organic Foods are Rich in Organic Minerals!

molecule. Every mineral contributes a unique factor to vitality, which is the positive proof of good health.

Organic whole grains contain all the essential parts and naturally-occurring nutrients of the entire grain seed. – See web: WholeGrainsCouncil.org

Beets and Celery for Longevity

Organic raw beets and celery have the highest amounts of organic sodium. We eat them almost daily, raw in salads and our fresh juices. Once a week we make a beet – veggie combination soup, based on traditional Russian Borscht. We know you'll like this recipe!

BRAGG HEARTY BEET – VEGGIE SOUP
Delicious Hot or Cold

1 ½ qts distilled water	2 unpeeled potatoes, dice
2 cups cabbage, slice	3 cups raw beets, shred
1 cup carrots, shred	1 cup celery, dice
2-3 garlic cloves, mince	1 tsp coconut aminos
1 small onion, mince	2 Tbsps organic olive oil
⅓ tsp No-Salt seasoning	1 tsp organic apple cider vinegar
3 fresh tomatoes (or 1 cup unsalted canned organic tomatoes)	

Mince onion, lightly saute in olive oil 3 minutes. Add 1½ quarts distilled water and coarsely shred veggies. Simmer in covered pot 15 minutes or until veggies are tender. Add tomatoes last 5 minutes. Season with coconut aminos, seasonings and organic apple cider vinegar just before serving. You can vary this recipe by adding other fresh organic veggies in season, and precooked lentils, brown rice, beans or lima beans. Serves 4 to 6.

107

As researchers in nutrition and longevity, we have been keenly interested in the long-lived people in Russia and the Ukraine. *"The Miracle of Fasting" is the #1 Health Book in Russia and Ukraine for over 40 years.* My father made several expeditions to primitive Russia and found people who lived amazingly long lives – some over 120 years! Beets were an important part of their daily diet. They got watercress from fresh mountain streams which they mixed with raw grated beets for a healthy salad!

Dad found areas where the main sources of water for drinking were rain and snow waters (distilled by Mother Nature) which helped reduce chances of having hardened arteries from inorganic minerals and chemical buildups.

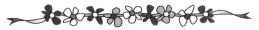

Soup rejoices the stomach, and prepares it to receive and digest other foods. – Jean Anthelme Brillat-Savarin

To err is human. Admit your faults, make amends, forgive yourself and learn from your mistakes. It's a wise person who also learns from the mistakes of others.

Many of these rural, ageless Russians had never tasted common table salt. Their arteries were healthy, flexible, youthful and free from the artery cloggers – inorganic minerals and chemical encrustations!

Salt is a Slow But Sure Killer!

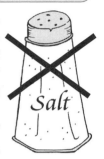

Common table salt (inorganic sodium chloride) is both unnecessary and injurious to the human body. It acts like the inorganic minerals found in almost all drinking water except steam-produced distilled water. Table salt can cause encrustations in the arteries, veins and capillaries. It can waterlog body tissues, making them flabby and without skin or muscle tone.

As a general rule, table salt users have a high elevation of blood pressure. According to medical statistics, the Japanese suffer from some of the highest blood pressure in the world. They are known to be the world's highest salt consumers. And my father's grandfather, who had a massive stroke in front of Dad's eyes at the dinner table, was a heavy user of inorganic salt. He put table salt on almost everything he ate – including tomatoes, watermelon, cantaloupe, celery and radishes – and he ate many salty foods, including ham, bacon, corned beef, hot dogs, luncheon meats, salted popcorn, pretzels and salted nuts.

Eating such large amounts of salt and salty foods gave him an unquenchable thirst. My dad would often watch his grandfather consume as many as 2 pitchers of water at each meal! He used table salt, ate salty foods and washed everything down with hard well water that was saturated with inorganic minerals. Is it any wonder that his arteries turned to stone and a stroke killed him?

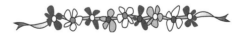

Shake your salt habit! Studies show the salt habit raises risk of heart attack, stroke, hypertension, kidney disease and stomach cancer.
– National Academy of Medicine – www.nam.edu

Desire for salty foods is an acquired taste. Your tastebuds can be retrained to appreciate natural flavors of foods. – Neal Barnard, M.D., "Food for Life"

Heavy Salt Intake Hastens Premature Death

The Chinese are now known as the world's highest consumers of table salt (inorganic salt – sodium chloride) with adults consistently consuming on average above 10g of salt a day!

Americans are not far behind the Chinese in the consumption of salt. Not only do Americans add plenty of salt to their foods, they also eat large amounts of ham, bacon, hot dogs, luncheon meats, corned beef, potato chips, salted nuts and many other foods with high concentrations of salt. No wonder heart disease is the #1 killer in America! Even people in their 30s and 40s suffer from high blood pressure, kidney trouble, arthritis and the greatest of all killers – arteriosclerosis – the clogging of the arteries, veins and blood vessels! The proper amount and the right kind of water helps to keep cholesterol levels down.

Organic Sodium – Powerful Natural Solvent

Organic sodium is a powerful natural solvent and neutralizer of toxic waste products. In contrast, table salt – an inorganic sodium chloride – not only is unnecessary, but is harmful to the body's chemistry.

In animal and human processes, organic sodium has many important functions. For the transmission of the electric induction current, which is generated in the nerve spirals by iron in the blood, a sodium liquid is necessary (as is shown by the construction of electric batteries). For this purpose, the normal blood serum contains a comparatively large quantity of organic sodium which favors and sustains the generation and conduction of the body's important and vital electric currents.

Moreover, organic sodium plays an important part in the formation of saliva, pancreatic juice and bile. The dissolving and reducing properties of sodium can be very distinctly recognized in the emulsification and the saponification of fats, especially in the bile. Organic sodium is a fat fighter. It helps to keep the waxy killer, cholesterol, at healthier levels of 150 to 180.

Enjoy healthy, organic foods for their wonderful abundance of life energy.

Organic sodium is essential for purifying the system of carbonaceous waste products. Let us remind you again that sodium is of value to the body only when obtained in its organic form from fruits, vegetables and kelp, etc!

As previously noted, inorganic salt is indigestible and especially when eaten in large quantities is not easily eliminated from the body. It is therefore deposited in the tissues of the body and an insatiable craving for water develops as the body attempts to wash the salt from its system. Thus the tissues and the vital organs become waterlogged. When this condition reaches the heart, we have what is known as congestive heart failure. The heart cannot function under the combined stress from hardened arteries, added to the flabbiness from body waterlogging. Congestive heart failure sadly kills millions every year!

Misinformation About Killer Salt

Using common table salt is one of the most twisted, widespread habits and is injurious to your health! The consumption of salt in the United States now amounts to more than 100 pounds per person each year, and its use is constantly increasing! The salt companies do a thorough brainwashing job, even telling people they need iodized salt to prevent goiters. Sodium chloride, or common table salt, is an inorganic substance which has been the subject of much confusion in the minds of people for many years – particularly in regard to its necessity as an adjunct to our food.

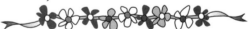

The American Heart Association says that daily sodium intake should be less than 2,400 milligrams per day, which is about 1¼ teaspoons of sodium chloride (table salt – inorganic sodium). We recommend using NO table salt. Throwing away the salt shaker is a positive step towards living The Bragg Healthy Lifestyle! Get your natural organic sodium from natural healthy foods.

The eating of much flesh fills us with a multitude of evil diseases and multitudes of evil desires. – Porphyry Malchus, Greek Philosopher, 233 A.D.

It's a little known fact that about 80% of sodium we eat comes not from salt we add at the table or during cooking, but from processed, packaged foods, canned, frozen and bakery products, etc. – Tufts University Nutrition Letter

Thy food shall be thy remedy. – Hippocrates, Father of Medicine, 400 B.C.

We Constantly Hear These False, Erroneous Statements About Salt:

- "The salt desire is instinctive to humans and animals."
- "It is the only substance which we take into our bodies directly from mineral elements."
- "Common table salt is one of the most essential of the mineral constituents of the body."
- "In hot weather, when we sweat a great deal, we lose the salt from our bodies. Therefore we should use large amounts of salt and salt tablets to replace it; or else we get sick, weak and suffer from exhaustion."
- "Without salt, we would die!"
- "When salt is entirely withheld from an animal, death from salt starvation ensues."

Salt – Harmful Preservative – Don't Use It!

All these assertions, and similar ones, are diametrically opposed to the truth! Why should sodium chloride be an exception among the other inorganic minerals?

111

Salt has been used in the human diet for thousand of years – but not because the human body needs it! **Salt was the first food preservative discovered by man.** Salt is still used extensively in the preservation of nearly all foods, especially meats and cheeses. It is found in baby foods, canned vegetables, canned fish, prepared cereals, all commercial breads and bakery goods. In fact, it is very hard to find any foods in the supermarkets that have not been contaminated with salt! Even in this modern age of refrigeration and other mechanical marvels, man still craves this primitive use of salt which was used to preserve and lengthen the shelf life of his food – and consequently shortens his own!

The salt eating habit is not instinctive! It is acquired, as are the other health-destroying and life-shortening, unhealthy habits, such as alcohol, smoking, coffee, drugs, etc. The taste or craving for salt is artificial, because salt paralyzes the 260 taste buds in the mouth. Like any other addiction, salt creates an unnatural craving by deadening certain warning signals of the body.

The advocates of salt point to the animals who often travel miles to the so-called "salt licks." My father studied some of the natural "salt lick" deposits and, on close examination, found little or no sodium!

Cattle, like humans, do not need inorganic sodium. When cattle are fed herbage grown in soils that are poor in mineral elements – especially sodium – such as mountain slopes where rains have carried away the most soluble parts of the soil and deposited them in valleys, they may try to satisfy this deficiency at an artificial (inorganic) "salt-lick."

An animal's taste buds, just like a human's, can be perverted by salt. Often a salt block is put in the pasture so the cattle will lick it, become excessively thirsty and consume large amounts of water. As in humans, the result is waterlogged tissues. Consequently, the cattle ranchers gain profit from waterlogged tissue weight when the cattle are brought to market. Remember, when you eat commercial meat, it may be saturated with inorganic salt, plus other toxins, hormones, drugs, etc. Please don't make matters worse by adding more table salt to it! See *mad-cow.org*

Plenty of fresh fruits, vegetables, seaweeds and salads in your diet will supply your body with all the organic sodium it needs. *For your healthy liquids you will find no purer drink than the juice of delicious, fresh organic fruits and vegetables and pure distilled water.*

Salt (Inorganic Sodium) is a Health Wrecker

Excessive use of inorganic sodium chloride (salt) and salty foods, leads to waterlogged humans. You often see young children 7 to 10 years and older who are so waterlogged that they have grotesque, bloated and prematurely old looking bodies. Just compare them to adults with bloated and puffed-up faces, arms, bellies, legs, ankles and feet. Please don't let this happen to you!

Stomach pains, migraines, allergies, asthma, angina, arthritis, back and joint pains; may all be symptoms of severe dehydration – which can easily be helped by drinking 8 glasses of distilled water daily and add 2 tsps organic apple cider vinegar and honey equally to 3 of them. Start increasing your water intake! Play it Safe – Be Water Wise and Health Safe!
– Paul C. Bragg, N.D., Ph.D., Originator of Health Stores

The "Fad" of Drinking Sea Water

From time to time during the past 85 years, some so-called "health experts" have advised drinking sea water to get the minerals which the body requires. They give the argument that billions of tons of top soil are washed into the ocean every year, and that the minerals from this rich soil can be absorbed by the human body to gain more health. Nothing could be farther from the truth! Yes, the ocean is a vast storehouse of inorganic minerals. But again we must positively state that the human body cannot absorb or utilize any inorganic mineral – whether it comes from a well, spring, river, lake or ocean. Then, too, ocean water has a very high concentration of inorganic sodium chloride (common table salt) which cannot be used by the body chemistry.

Don't drink sea water, no matter what you have been told or read! Sailors and shipwrecked people have tried it, and they had an agonizing death!

Sea Salt is Inorganic Sodium (Salt)!

Due to all of the bad publicity about table salt in recent years, many health food stores and manufacturers have begun promoting the use of sea salt. Their rationalization is that this particular form of sodium is healthy and natural since it is coming from the sea. Well, one could make the same argument for common table salt that is taken from the earth via a quarry!

The bottom line is this – no matter where or how on earth it comes from, if salt is not first transformed by plants from inorganic sodium into organic sodium, it can't be properly absorbed into the body! If you enjoy the taste of salt on food, it's healthiest to come from a plant source. A healthy option is to sprinkle powdered kelp over food which Dad helped bring to the market over 60 years ago.

The body is self-cleansing and self-healing! It is our duty if we want vibrant, glorious health, to do all we can to make the body work efficiently to maintain vital, super health. Not only is a healthy diet necessary, but so are good sleeping habits, outdoor physical activity, deep breathing and a serene, peaceful mind. We cannot live by bread alone. We must have spiritual food. Also strive for a perfect healthy balance: physical, mental, emotional and spiritual!

Sea Kelp – Rich Organic Minerals from the Sea

When you eat sea plants such as kelp and seaweed you are following the rules of scientific nutrition. The sea vegetation converts the inorganic minerals of the sea into organic minerals, and there are many kinds of sea vegetables to enjoy. Try Bladderwack, Dulse, Irish Moss, Rockweed or Sea Lettuce (visit: *SeaVeg.com*). We sprinkle kelp on our salads and other foods. It gives food a tangy flavor and at the same time furnishes the body with natural organic iodine, potassium, calcium and magnesium. Plus we enjoy various seaweeds flattened out as bread with salads. We also roll mashed avocado, etc. in seaweed – it's delicious.

Overweight, Obesity and Edema

Long before the stage of congestive heart failure is reached, the excessive salt eater suffers from many miseries. The most common of these are being overweight and obese. **Statistics show that 65% of Americans are overweight** – and not all of this is excess fat! Many times being overweight is caused by waterlogged tissues. This overweight problem will continue as long as these people use salt on their foods, and especially if they partake freely of salted foods such as canned fish, salted butter, ham, bacon, canned vegetables, cheese, luncheon meats, frozen foods, salted popcorn and nuts. Like hard water, this salt-filled diet damages the arteries, veins and capillaries, as well as the internal organs and tissues of the body.

114

ARE YOU OVERWEIGHT OR OBESE? A person is considered to be overweight if they are 10 or more pounds above the normal weight for their sex and height; 20% or more above the normal weight is obese. Overweight and obesity are both labels for weight ranges that are more than what is considered healthy for a given height. The terms also identify weight ranges that have been shown to increase the likelihood of diseases and other health problems. – cdc.gov/obesity

---

Iodine is a health-promoting trace element essential for life. Its primary biological role lies in the production of the thyroid hormones. Iodine happens to be found abundantly in sea vegetables and plants.

God makes all things good; man often meddles with them and they can become evil. – Rousseau

The kidneys are the organs most severely affected by the salt-eating habit. They become weakened and unable to eliminate this large amount of salt, which is then retained in the tissues where, of course, it must be held in solution by water. This condition produces edema, which generally occurs in tandem with kidney disease and cirrhosis of the liver.

"Edema" is a common disease of the unhealthy in America. Observe the ankles and legs of the average obese person, all too often swollen and puffed-up. This condition is sometimes so severe that their ankles must be bandaged before the afflicted person can stand up. In time, edema becomes chronic and interferes with circulation to such a degree that leg ulcers or gangrene set in and an amputation might become necessary.

There are no body organs so mercilessly mistreated as the kidneys and liver! Think of the gallons of toxic water saturated with inorganic minerals, chloride and fluoride which these organs try to neutralize! Not only in the water that we drink by itself, but water mixed with coffee, tea, alcohol, colas and other soft drinks, plus canned, frozen foods, catsup, mustard and other seasonings with high salt concentrations. Our poor kidneys and liver! What a terrible beating they take! No wonder millions sicken and die long before their time. Man doesn't die: he kills himself by his faulty, unthinking and unhealthy lifestyle!

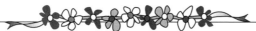

Don't procrastinate and keep waiting for "the right moment."
Today – take action, plan, plot and follow through with your goals, dreams and healthy lifestyle living! You will be a winner in life when you Captain your life to success! – Patricia Bragg

Edema: is observable swelling from fluid accumulation in body tissues. Edema most commonly occurs in the feet and legs. Edema can be isolated to a small area or affect the entire body. It an be the result of medication or an underlying disease – often heart failure, kidney disease or cirrhosis. When your body, legs, ankles and feet swell, your heart cannot function correctly and becomes burdened and unhealthy! – Mayo Clinic

The Bragg Healthy Lifestyle Promotes Super Health and Longevity

The Bragg Healthy Lifestyle consists of eating a diet of 60% to 70% fresh, live, organically grown foods; raw vegetables, salads, fresh fruits and juices; sprouts, raw seeds and raw nuts; all-natural 100% whole-grain breads, pastas, cereals and nutritious beans and legumes. These are the no cholesterol, no fat, no salt, "live foods" which combine to make up the body fuel that creates healthy, lively people that want to exercise and be fit. This healthy

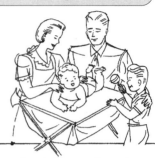

When babies are brought up on and taught to live The Bragg Healthy Lifestyle, they can enjoy longer lives in painless, tireless and ageless bodies!

diet also creates energy. This is the reason people become revitalized and reborn into a fresh new life filled with joy, health, vitality, youthfulness and longevity! There are millions of healthy Bragg followers around the world proving that this Bragg Healthy Lifestyle works!

The World's Greatest Health Secret

The "secret" of health lies in **internal cleanliness!** To be 100% healthy, a body must be free from deposits of inorganic minerals that come from drinking city tap water and waters from lakes, rivers, wells and springs. The body is contaminated by inorganic minerals from these sources. Encrustations form that clog and obstruct the body's pipes and impair the vital organs.

The body needs absolutely pure H_2O. Water that comes from raw, organically grown fruits and vegetables is the best life-giving water. It is water that has been charged with solar energy, health-building vitamins, organic minerals and marvelous enzymes! Enzymes can help you build up a natural resistance to any ailment as they help to flush out the accumulated deposits of inorganic minerals and work to dissolve the toxins that are buried deep in your tissues and organs.

Nourish the mind like you would your body.
The mind cannot survive on junk food! – Jim Rohn

Good Elimination is Vital to Health

Studies reveal the presence of toxic poisons in cases of constipation. When these toxins are absorbed into the general circulation, the liver "your detoxifying organ" is unable to cope with them. These toxins are then thrown back into the body to cause degenerative diseases, toxemia, cancer, premature ageing, sickness and lack of energy.

Your lifestyle and diet play a vital role in the maintenance of health, good elimination and the prevention of disease. Research shows that diets composed of refined white flour and sugar; preserved meats, such as hot dogs and luncheon meats; white rice; coffee, tea, cola drinks and all alcohol; margarine; overcooked vegetables; high fat, sugared, salted, and processed foods create serious health problems, especially in the colon and intestinal tract, heart and respiratory areas. It's wise to never eat refined, processed, embalmed and dead, unhealthy foods!!!

For Easier Flowing Bowel Movements

It's natural to squat to have bowel movements. It opens up your anal area more directly. When on a toilet, putting feet up 6-8" on waste basket or footstool gives the same squatting effect. Now raise arms, stretch hands above head so the transverse colon can empty and roll out completely with ease. It's important for you to drink 8-10 glasses pure water daily – works miracles! After the dinner meal take one psyllium husk vegetarian capsule daily.

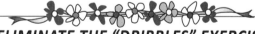

ELIMINATE THE "DRIBBLES" EXERCISE:
To keep bladder and sphincter muscles tight and toned, urinate – stop – urinate – stop, 4 times, twice daily when voiding, especially after age 40. This simple exercise works wonders for both men and women!

The World Health Organization reports that some 31 million people worldwide – are victims of 4 chronic conditions linked to unhealthy lifestyles: circulatory diseases (especially heart attacks and strokes), diabetes, cancer and respiratory disease! – www.who.int

Pure water, the natural solvent of the body, regulates all body functions, including the eliminations of toxins and body waste.

Organic Fresh Juices are the Magic Cleansers

The raw juices of organic fruits and vegetables are internal cleansers and blood purifiers. These are what we call "the waters of perpetual health and youthfulness." The rays of the sun send billions of atoms into plant life. We can use this solar energy to attain vigorous health, unlimited vitality and physical endurance.

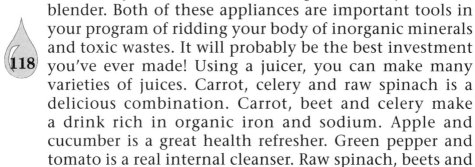 The miracle organic fruits and vegetables from solar energy can fight accumulation of inorganic minerals and toxic poisons you have allowed to be deposited in your body. Fruit and vegetable juices are natural detergents for the human body. Try to get a quart or more of freshly-squeezed fruit and vegetable juices into your body every day.

Go to your Health Store and purchase a juicer and blender. Both of these appliances are important tools in your program of ridding your body of inorganic minerals and toxic wastes. It will probably be the best investment you've ever made! Using a juicer, you can make many varieties of juices. Carrot, celery and raw spinach is a delicious combination. Carrot, beet and celery make a drink rich in organic iron and sodium. Apple and cucumber is a great health refresher. Green pepper and tomato is a real internal cleanser. Raw spinach, beets and watercress will flood your bloodstream with organic iron. Parsley, celery and carrot juiced together is a delicious, healthy combination. Cabbage juice (Stanford University Medical School discovered it helps heal ulcers), onion, garlic, pea-pods, turnip-tops, lettuce, kale, dandelion and endive juices are all packed with vital solar energy, vitamins, organic minerals, trace minerals and enzymes.

Fruit juices play an important role in building a clean, healthy bloodstream and energized body. Organic apple, pineapple, cherry, blackberry, orange, grapefruit, and prune juices are the "nectar of the gods" for you to enjoy.

Healthy, healing dietary fibers are found in fresh organic vegetables, fresh fruits, salads and whole grains and their products. These health-builders help to normalize blood pressure, weight and cholesterol levels and promotes healthy elimination and super health.

Chapter 8

Choose Your Foods Wisely

Let Natural Food Be Your Medicine

What does food really do in the human body? What relationship does it have with long life and vigorous health – and to disease, misery and physical suffering? How can it be of influence in cleansing the body of inorganic minerals and toxic poisons? We must have a fundamental, deep understanding of these questions before we can fully appreciate the role diet plays in the health maintenance of the living processes, the prevention of human diseases, and the restoration of health and the prolongation of life.

A balanced diet gives the body nourishment, energy and power. It's made up of 60% to 70% organic raw fruit and vegetables; 20% protein from vegetable sources (see page 125) and equal parts of natural sugars (honey, stevia), natural starches (whole grains, brown rice, etc.), and unsaturated fats (organic olive oil, soy or flaxseed oils). This balanced diet puts your body on the alkaline side and helps to keep the body internally cleaner.

119

Healthy Plant-Based Daily Food Guide

Be a Health Crusader – copy and share with friends, clubs, etc.

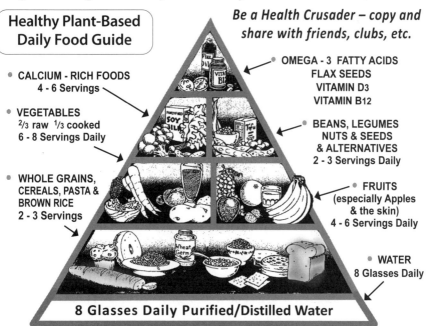

- OMEGA - 3 FATTY ACIDS
  FLAX SEEDS
  VITAMIN D3
  VITAMIN B12

- CALCIUM - RICH FOODS
  4 - 6 Servings

- VEGETABLES
  2/3 raw 1/3 cooked
  6 - 8 Servings Daily

- BEANS, LEGUMES
  NUTS & SEEDS
  & ALTERNATIVES
  2 - 3 Servings Daily

- WHOLE GRAINS,
  CEREALS, PASTA &
  BROWN RICE
  2 - 3 Servings

- FRUITS
  (especially Apples
  & the skin)
  4 - 6 Servings Daily

- WATER
  8 Glasses Daily

8 Glasses Daily Purified/Distilled Water

You are what you eat, drink, breathe, think, say and do!
Patricia Bragg, Pioneer Health Crusader

Start Eating Healthy Foods For Super Energy

This *Healthy Plant-Based Daily Food Guide Pyramid* illustration represents a more ideal way of eating for achieving optimal nutrition, health and wellness. You will notice that this Food Guide Pyramid is based on healthy organic plant foods, with emphasis on pure water, fruits, vegetables, whole grains, vegetable protein foods, non-dairy calcium foods, and raw nuts and seeds. Eating a diet based on these dietary guidelines will help you get the nutrients needed for optimal health. It's not only the best type of diet for wellness, disease prevention and longevity, it also provides the right balance for building a healthy nervous system.

Purified/Distilled Water: At the pyramid's foundation is purified water. We recommend drinking *pure distilled water* as it is the best water for the body! ***Drink at least eight – 8 oz glasses of distilled water daily and even more if your lifestyle (sports, work, etc.) requires it.***

Whole Grains: Whole grains are the next level of the pyramid. Avoid all processed, refined grain products and eat only unrefined, organic whole grain bread and cereal products. Grains such as whole wheat, brown rice, oats, millet, quinoa, as well as 100% whole grain breads and cereals are the best. One serving of whole grains is equal to 1 slice whole grain bread, 1 ounce ready-to-eat whole grain cereal, 1 cup cooked whole grains such as brown rice, oatmeal or other grains, 1 cup 100% whole wheat (or other whole grains) pasta or noodles, and 1 ounce of other whole grain products. ***We recommend eating 2-3 servings of organic, non-GMO whole grains daily.***

Vegetables: We recommend eating as many of your vegetables organic and raw (uncooked, in salads, juices, etc.) as possible! When you cook vegetables, do not overcook them. Steaming or lightly stir-frying is best.

I now live on legumes, vegetables and fruits. No dairy, no meat of any kind, no chicken, no turkey, and very little fish, only once in a while. It changed my metabolism and I lost 24 pounds. I did research and found 82% of people who go on a plant-based diet begin to heal themselves, as I did.
– Bill Clinton, United States President, 1993-2001

It's magnificent to live long, if one keeps healthy and fit. – Harry Fosdick

The more colorful rainbow of vegetables you eat, the better they are for your health as they contain more valuable nutrients and healthful phytonutrients. Eat a wide variety of organic vegetables daily. One vegetable serving is equal to 1 cup cooked vegetables or 1 cup raw uncooked vegetables, 1 cup salad, or ¾ cup vegetable juice. *We recommend having 6-8 or more vegetable servings daily.*

Fruits: Like vegetables, the more colorful the fruits the better they are for you. Enjoy organic fruits as much as possible! One serving of fruit is equal to 1 medium apple, banana, orange, pear or other fruit, ½ cup fruit, ½ cup of fruit juice or ¼ cup dried fruit. *We recommend eating 4-6 servings or more of organic fruits daily.*

Calcium-Rich Foods: These are plant-derived calcium-rich foods. Plant source of calcium are healthier than dairy products because they do not contain saturated fats or cholesterol. Health calcium-rich foods contain foods such as oat milk, tofu, broccoli and green leafy vegetables. Examples of serving sizes of plant-derived calcium-rich foods include: 1 cup oat milk, ½ cup tofu, ⅓ cup almonds, 1 cup cooked or 2 cups of high calcium raw greens (kale, collards, broccoli, bok choy or other Chinese greens), 1 cup of calcium-rich beans (e.g. soy, white, navy, Great Northern), ½ cup seaweed, 1 tablespoon blackstrap molasses, 5 or more figs. *We recommend having 4-6 servings of healthy non-dairy sources of calcium rich foods daily, see page 127.*

121

Beans, Legumes, Nuts & Seeds: This group are the healthy protein foods. Vegetable protein foods are more optimal compared to animal protein foods. Vegetable proteins do not contain the artery clogging saturated fats and cholesterol found in animal foods. They also contain protective factors to prevent heart disease, cancer and diabetes. Vegetable proteins are high quality and provide the body with the essential amino acids that it requires. One serving of vegetable protein foods include: 1 cup cooked legumes (beans, lentils, dried peas), ½ cup firm tofu or tempeh, 1 serving of "veggie meat" alternate (e.g. veggie burger patty), 3 tablespoons nut or seed butter, 1 cup almond or rice milk. *We recommend you have 2-3 or more vegetable protein servings daily with meals.*

Healthy Fats, Essential Fatty Acids, Omega-3 and Other Nutrients: Servings of healthy fats include: 1 teaspoon flaxseed oil, 1 tablespoon of organic extra-virgin olive oil, 3 tablespoons raw walnuts. Other healthy essentials at the top include ground flaxseed and nutritional B-Complex supplements that provide vitamin B12, including nutritional yeast. Do provide your body with nutritional supplements your body requires for optimal health and longevity!

Start Health Educating Your Taste Buds

It will take strong willpower to change old habits of eating the average dead foods to eating healthy, live foods. For a while there will be a craving for the unhealthy foods which you have probably eaten most of your life. But if you are positive in your selection of natural foods, soon the old desire for devitalized foods will leave you!

In time, you will find an added pleasure in enjoying the true tastes of the healthy, live foods you eat! You will be able to discern when your 260 taste buds have recovered from salt paralysis and have come alive again!

Eliminating Meat is Healthiest

Most uninformed nutritionists call meat the #1 source of protein. Those proteins coming from the vegetable kingdom are referred to as the #2 proteins. This is a sad and terrible mistake. It should be the other way around!

In this day and age, almost all meat is laden with herbicides, fungicides, pesticides and other chemicals that are sprayed on or poured into the feed which these animals consume! They are also pumped full of hormones, antibiotics, growth stimulators and all kinds of drugs to fatten them up and keep them from dying from the extremely unhealthy conditions most of them live in! This is not to mention the admitted fact many of them are fed dead, ground up carcasses of other feed lot fallen animals who, for a variety of reasons, did not make it to the slaughterhouse (visit: *www.mad-cow.org*).

Evidence shows that eating a meat based diet is bad for the environment, aggravates global hunger, brutalizes animals and compromises your health.

Speaking of the horrors of the slaughterhouses, what kind of chemical reaction do you suppose would occur in your body if somebody put a choke chain around your neck to keep you in line, shoved you onto a conveyor belt, and made you watch in horror as all of those in line in front of you were beheaded one by one? Well, your body would be pumped so full of adrenaline from all that fear you wouldn't know what hit you! Unused adrenaline is extremely toxic. If you think for a minute that most of the meat that you consume is not packed with this toxic substance, you're sadly mistaken!

Also, consider the fact that cattle, sheep, chickens, etc., are all vegetarians. When you eat them, you are just eating polluted vegetables. Why not skip all the waste and toxins and just eat healthy, organic vegetables?

And what about that myth that you have to eat meat to get your protein? If that were true, where do you suppose farm animals, especially horses, get their protein? They are vegetarians! They get their protein from the grains and grasses that they eat. You are no different. You can get all the proteins you need, and then some, from the organic grains, nuts, seeds, beans, fruits and vegetables on this planet for you to enjoy eating to stay healthy (see chart page 125).

123

Meat is also a major source of toxic uric acid and cholesterol, both harmful to your health. If you are going to include meat in your diet, it should not be eaten more than 2 times a week. In our opinion, fresh fish can be the least toxic of the flesh proteins. But beware of fish from polluted waters! They can be loaded with mercury, lead, cadmium, DDT and many other toxic substances. If you are unable to test the waters from where your fish come, don't risk eating them! And avoid shellfish – shrimp, lobster and crayfish. They are garbage-eating bottom-feeders – the rats and flies of the water kingdom. They eat all of the rotting, decaying scum and refuse off the bottoms of the oceans, lakes and rivers. Next come chicken and turkey (never eat the skin, which is heavy in cholesterol). Third place goes to lamb and beef.

No man can violate Nature's Laws and escape her penalties! – Julian Johnson

People should not eat pork or pork products. The pig is the only animal besides man that develops arteriosclerosis or hardening of the arteries. In fact, this animal is so loaded with cholesterol that in cold weather, unprotected pigs and hogs will become solid and stiff, as though frozen solid. Also, this animal is often infected with a dangerous parasite which causes trichinosis.

We enjoy being vegetarians and not polluting our bodies with unhealthy, meat, fowl and fish proteins! *We feel it's safer and healthier getting our proteins from organic vegetables, beans, legumes, nuts, seeds, etc.*

Over–Fueling the Body is a Slow Killer!

Some people eat as though they were going to do the hardest kind of physical labor! A sedentary person – by habit and conditioning – will get up in the morning and eat a heavy breakfast of cooked or dry cereal, hot cakes with bacon, eggs, buttered toast and a stimulating beverage like black tea or coffee. These same people then go to work in an office, store, etc., and sit or stand around all day. They will usually have mid-morning snacks and then at noon they will eat a heavy meal: bread, meat, a dessert and a beverage like a sugared soft drink or coffee. In the mid-afternoon they again have snacks and more sugared drinks. Then at home they have their biggest meal of the day; consisting of meat, potatoes, bread, dessert and a beverage. Typically they end their day watching TV – while eating another snack! This kind of daily habitual over-eating is making millions of sick, fat, exhausted people. This habit is sending them to doctors, clinics, hospitals and too many to an early grave! Sad Facts: millions are sick and grossly overweight and it's all due to unhealthy lifestyle habits.

The person living the average, inactive life can't possibly burn up these large amounts of food! So what happens to people who eat this way? You know as well as we do that they are sick or half-sick for most of their entire lives. They fill the doctors' offices, pharmacies and hospitals with all their health problems brought on by their unhealthy lifestyles. Millions more end up in old people's homes, convalescent and mental facilities.

Plant-Based Protein Chart

BEANS & LEGUMES	PROTEIN
(1 cup cooked)	IN GRAMS
Soybeans	29
Lentils	18
Adzuki Beans.	17
Cannellini	17
Navy Beans	16
Split Peas	16
Black Beans	15
Garbanzos (chick peas) . .	15
Kidney Beans.	15
Great Northern Beans . . .	15
Lima Beans	15
Black-eyed Peas	14
Pinto Beans	14
Mung Beans.	14
Tofu (3 oz.)	7 to 12
Green Peas (whole)	9

VEGETABLES	PROTEIN
(1 Serving or 1 cup)	IN GRAMS
Spirulina	.8.6
Corn (1 cob)	5
Potato (with skin)	5
Mushrooms, Oyster.	5
Artichoke (1 medium). . . .	4
Collard Greens	4
Broccoli	4
Brussel Sprouts	4
Mushrooms, Shiitake . .	3.5
Swiss Chard.	3
Kale	.2.5
Asparagus (5 spears)	2
String Beans.	2
Beets	2
Peas	2
Sweet Potato	3
Summer Squash.	2
Cabbage.	2
Carrot	2
Cauliflower	2
Squash	2
Celery	1
Spinach	1
Bell Peppers.	1
Cucumber	1
Eggplant	1
Leeks	1
Lettuce.	1
Tomato (1 medium)	1
Radish	1
Turnips	1

FRUITS	PROTEIN
(1 Serving or 1 cup)	IN GRAMS
Avocado (1 medium).	4
Banana (1).	1 to 2
Blackberries (1 cup).	2
Pomegranate (1)	1.5
Blueberries (1 cup)	1
Cantaloupe (1 cup)	1
Cherries (1 cup).	1
Grapes (1 cup)	1
Honeydew (1 cup)	1
Kiwi (1 large)	1
Lemon (1)	1
Mango (1)	1
Nectarine (1)	1
Orange (1)	1
Peach (1)	1
Pear (1)	1
Pineapple (1 cup)	1
Plum (1).	1
Raspberries (1 cup)	1
Strawberries (1 cup).	1
Watermelon (1 cup)	1

RAW NUTS & SEEDS	PROTEIN
(1/4 cup or 4 Tbsps)	IN GRAMS
Chia Seeds.	12
Macadamia Nuts	11
Flax Seeds	8
Sunflower Seeds.	8
Almonds	7
Pumpkin Seeds	7
Sesame Seeds.	7
Walnuts.	5
Brazil Nuts.	5
Hazelnuts	5
Pine Nuts.	4
Cashews.	4

GRAINS & RICE	PROTEIN
(1 cup cooked)	IN GRAMS
Triticale	25
Millet.	.8.4
Amaranth	7
Oat Bran	7
Wild Rice.	7
Couscous (whole wheat). .	6
Bulgur Wheat	6
Buckwheat.	6
Teff.	6
Oat Groats.	6
Barley.	5
Quinoa	5
Brown Rice	5
Spelt.	5

NUT BUTTERS	PROTEIN
(2 Tbsps)	IN GRAMS
Peanut Butter	7 to 9
Almond Butter	5 to 8
Cashew Butter.	4 to 5
Sesame - Tahini	6

DAIRY & NUT MILKS	PROTEIN
(1 cup)	IN GRAMS
Oat Milk	.3 to 4
Almond Milk.	1 to 2
Rice Milk	1
Eggs (1) *(free-range)*	6

125

This chart displays protein content of common vegetarian foods.
Note that in order to determine amount of protein that is optimal for your body, use the following formula that is based on a vegan diet: *RDA recommends that we take in 0.36 grams of protein per pound that we weigh* (100 lbs. x 0.36 = 36 grams).

Data from webs: *TheHolyKale.com • VegParadise.com • vrg.org (Vegetarian Resource Group).*

Warnings on Milk and It's Dangers!

We do not recommend using animal milks, specifically cow's milk, for several reasons. First, almost all milk is pasteurized (boiled). Milk that is not labeled raw has been boiled to kill all bacteria so you don't get sick from drinking it. Bacteria is not the only thing that is killed during boiling. Pasteurized milk is dead. If anything is left alive, the homogenization process destroys it. Why would you want to drink dead milk?

Milk also contains an enzyme called lactose which most people are allergic to. The major symptom of a lactose allergy is mucus formation. Many people think lots of mucus and handkerchiefs, nose-blowing and tissues are just a normal part of life. But they're not! These people haven't realized that they are lactose intolerant. If they stopped consuming milk and other dairy products, most would find themselves drastically reducing their mucus production and use of tissues.

126

Be informed and take into consideration all of the herbicides, pesticides and fungicides that cattle ingest through their feed. These toxins are passed on to you through their milk. This is to say nothing of all the hormones, growth stimulators, antibiotics and other drugs that are pumped into cattle to treat disease and increase their weight and milk production. These chemicals also make their way into the milk. As far as raw milk is concerned, remember the reason that pasteurization became mandated by law was because so many people were dying from bacterial diseases that they contracted from drinking raw milk.

And what about the cattle industry's policy of feeding cows the rendered (ground-up) remains of other cows? How healthy do you think the milk of a cannibal cow really is? Also, if you think these cattle are given distilled water to drink, you need to visit a feed lot and see for yourself. You would be appalled at the conditions! In short, if you value your health, switch to nut and rice milks, abstain from cow's milk and its products: cheese, buttermilk, sour cream, cream cheese, cream, butter, yogurt and ice cream.

Knowing these teachings gives true life & good health for you. – Proverbs 4:22

Benefit From Natural Foods Rich in Calcium

There are some very fine sources of calcium other than milk. We prefer the organic calcium found in kale, greens, corn, beans, vegetables, soybeans and tofu. Dr. Neal Barnard and Dr. Harold Lynch point out that all natural foods contain appreciable amounts of calcium. This chart below shows some of the many foods that contain large amounts of organic calcium you should include in your healthy diet.

Calcium Content of Some Common Foods

Food Source	mgs	Food Source	mgs
Almonds, 1 oz	80	Kale, (raw/steamed)	180
Artichokes, (raw/steamed)	51	Kohlrabi, (raw/steamed)	40
Beans, (kidney, pinto, red)	89	Mustard greens, 1 cup	138
Beans, (great northern, navy)	128	Oatmeal, 1 cup	120
Beans, (white)	161	Orange, 1 large	96
Blackstrap molasses, 1 Tbsp	137	Prunes, 4 whole	45
Bok choy, (raw/steamed)	158	Raisins, 4 oz.	45
Broccoli, (raw/steamed)	178	Rhubarb, (cooked) 1 cup	105
Brussels sprouts, (raw/steamed)	56	Rutabaga, (raw/steamed)	72
Buckwheat pancake	99	Sesame seeds (unhulled) 1 oz	381
Cabbage, (raw/steamed)	50	Spinach (raw/steamed)	244
Cauliflower, (raw/steamed)	34	Soybeans,	73
Collards, (raw/steamed)	152	Soymilk, fortified.	150
Corn tortilla	60	Tofu, firm.	258
Cornbread, 1 piece	28	Turnip greens, 1 cup	198
Figs, (5 medium)	135	Whole wheat bread, 1 slice	17

Sources: "Back to Eden", Jethro Kloss; "Health Nutrient Bible", Lynn Sonberg; website: vrg.org/nutrition/calcium.htm, chart by Brenda Davis, R.D.

Recommended Daily Intakes of Calcium

The amount of calcium required for bone health and to maintain adequate rates of calcium retention in a healthy body are: 0-6 months: 200 mg; 7-12 months: 260 mg; 1-3 years: 700 mg; 4-8 years: 1,000 mg; 9-18 years: 1,300 mg; 19-50 years: 1,000 mg; 51-70 years (men): 1,000 mg; 51-70 years (women): 1,200 mg; and 71+ years: 1,200 mg (developed by "Food & Nutrition Board" – *ods.od.nih.gov*)

> ***Read these 2 important books on milk and why to avoid milk:***
> • *"Mad Cows and Milk Gate" by Virgil Hulse M.D.*
> • *"Milk, the Deadly Poison" by Robert Cohen*
> *visit websites: www.NotMilk.com and www.pcrm.org*
> *(Physicians Committee for Responsible Medicine)*

Food and Product Summary

Today, many American foods are highly processed or refined, robbing them of essential nutrients, vitamins, minerals and enzymes. Many also contain harmful, toxic and dangerous chemicals (see lists of "Foods to Avoid" next page). The research findings and experience of top nutritionists, physicians and dentists have led to the discovery that devitalized foods are a major cause of poor health, illness, cancer and premature death. Scientific research has shown that most of these afflictions can be prevented and that once detected, can be arrested or even reversed through nutritional and healthy lifestyle methods.

Enjoy Super Health with Natural Foods

1. **RAW FOODS:** Fresh fruits and raw vegetables organically grown are always best. Enjoy nutritious variety garden salads with raw vegetables, sprouts, raw nuts and seeds.

2. **VEGETABLES and PROTEINS:**
   a. Legumes, lentils, brown rice, soybeans, and all beans.
   b. Nuts and seeds, raw and unsalted (lightly roasted okay).
   c. We prefer healthier vegetarian proteins. If you must have animal protein, then be sure it's hormone–free, and organically fed and no more than 1 or 2 times a week.
   d. Dairy products – fertile range-free eggs (not over 4 weekly), unprocessed hard cheese and feta goat's cheese. We choose not to use dairy products. Try the healthier non-dairy soy, rice, coconut, and almond milks and soy cheeses, delicious soy yogurt and soy and rice ice cream.

3. **FRUITS and VEGETABLES:** Organically grown is always best, grown without use of poisonous sprays and toxic chemical fertilizers. Urge markets to stock organic produce! Steam, bake, sauté and wok vegetables as short a time as possible to retain best nutritional content, flavor and use raw veggies in salads, sandwiches, etc. Also enjoy fresh juices.

4. **ORGANIC non-GMO WHOLE GRAIN CEREALS, BREADS & FLOURS:** They contain important B-Complex vitamins, vitamin E, minerals, fiber and the important unsaturated fatty acids.

5. **COLD or EXPELLER-PRESSED VEGETABLE OILS:** Organic first press extra virgin olive oil (is best), soy, sunflower, flax and sesame oils are excellent sources of healthy, essential, unsaturated fatty acids. We still use oils sparingly.

Avoid These Processed, Refined, Harmful Foods:

Once you realize the harm caused to your body by unhealthy refined, chemicalized, deficient foods, you'll want to eliminate "killer" foods:

- **Refined sugar / artificial sweeteners** (toxic aspartame) or their products such as jams, jellies, preserves, marmalades, yogurts, ice cream, sherbets, Jello, cake, candy, cookies, all chewing gum, colas and diet drinks, pies, pastries, and all sugared fruit juices and fruits canned in sugar syrup. (Health Stores have delicious healthy replacements, such as Stevia, raw honey, 100% maple syrup, and agave nectar, so seek and buy the best).

- **White flour products** such as white bread, wheat-white bread, enriched flours, rye bread that has white flour in it, dumplings, biscuits, buns, gravy, pasta, pancakes, waffles, soda crackers, pizza, ravioli, pies, pastries, cakes, cookies, prepared and commercial puddings and ready-mix bakery products. Most are made with dangerous (oxy-cholesterol) powdered milk and powdered eggs. (Health Stores have a variety of 100% non-GMO whole grain organic products, breads, chips, crackers, pastas, desserts).

- **Salted foods**, such as pretzels, corn chips, potato chips, crackers and nuts.

- **Refined white rice** and pearl barley. • **Fried fast foods.** • **Indian ghee**.

- **Refined dry processed cereals** that are sugared, such as cornflakes, etc.

- **Foods that contain Olestra**, palm and cottonseed oil.

- **Peanuts and peanut butter** that contain hydrogenated, hardened oils and any peanuts with mold and all molds that can cause allergies.

- **Margarine** – combines heart-deadly trans-fatty acids and saturated fats.

- **Saturated fats and hydrogenated oils** – enemies that clog the arteries.

- **Coffee, soft drinks, teas, alcohol, sugared juices** – even if decaffeinated.

- **Fresh pork / products.** • **Fried, fatty, greasy meats.** • **Irradiated GMO foods.**

- **Smoked meats**, such as ham, bacon, sausage and all smoked fish.

- **Luncheon meats**, hot dogs, salami, bologna, corned beef, pastrami and packaged meats containing dangerous sodium nitrate or nitrite.

- **Dried fruits** containing sulphur dioxide – a toxic preservative.

- **Chickens, turkeys and meats injected with hormones** or fed with commercial feed containing any drugs or toxins.

- **Canned soups** – read labels for sugar, salt, starch, flour and preservatives.

- **Foods containing preservatives, additives,** benzoate of soda, salt, sugar, cream of tartar, drugs, irradiated and genetically engineered foods.

- **Day-old cooked vegetables**, potatoes and pre-mixed, wilted lifeless salads.

- **All commercial vinegars:** pasteurized, filtered, distilled, white, malt and synthetic vinegars are dead vinegars! (We use only organic raw, unfiltered apple cider vinegar with the "Mother Enzyme" as used in olden times.)

Please follow The Bragg Healthy Lifestyle to provide the basic, healthy nourishment to maintain your precious health.

129

HEALTHY BEVERAGES
Fresh Juices, Herb Teas & Energy Drinks

These freshly squeezed organic vegetable and fruit juices are important to *The Bragg Healthy Lifestyle*. It's not wise to drink beverages with your main meals, as it dilutes the digestive juices. But it's great during the day to have a glass of freshly squeezed orange juice, grapefruit juice, vegetable juice, raw, organic apple cider vinegar drink (see below), or herbal tea – these are all ideal pick-me-up beverages.

Apple Cider Vinegar Drink – Mix 1-2 tsps. raw, organic apple cider vinegar (with the 'Mother' enzyme) and (optional) to taste raw honey or pure maple syrup *(if diabetic, to sweeten use 2 stevia drops)* in 8 oz. of distilled or purified water. Take glass upon arising, an hour before lunch and dinner.

Delicious Hot or Cold Cider Drink – Add 2-3 cinnamon sticks and 4 cloves to water and boil. Steep 20 minutes or more. Before serving add raw organic apple cider vinegar and sweetener to taste.

Bragg's Favorite Juice Drink – This drink consists of all raw vegetables *(remember organic is best)* which we prepare in our juicer / blender: carrots, celery, cucumber, beets, cabbage, tomatoes, watercress, kale, parsley, or any vegetable combination you prefer. The great purifier, garlic we enjoy, but it's optional.

Bragg's Favorite Healthy Energy Smoothie – After our morning stretch and exercises we often enjoy this drink instead of fruit. It's a delicious and powerfully nutritious meal anytime: lunch, dinner or in a thermos at work, school, the gym or during sports or hikes. You can freeze for popsicles too.

Bragg's Favorite Healthy Energy Smoothie

Prepare the following in a blender, add frozen juice cubes if desired colder; Choice of: freshly squeezed orange or grapefruit juice; carrot and greens juice; unsweetened pineapple juice; or 1^1/2 - 2 cups purified or distilled water with:

2 tsps spirulina or green powder
^{1}/3 tsp nutritional yeast
2 dates or prunes-pitted
1 "Emergen-C" Vitamin C packet
1 tsp protein powder (optional)

1-2 bananas or fresh fruit
1-2 tsps almond or nut butter
1 tsp flaxseed oil or grind seeds
1 tsp raw honey (optional)
^{1}/2 tsp lecithin granules

Optional: 4-6 apricots (sun-dried) soak in jar overnight in purified distilled water or unsweetened pineapple juice. We soak enough to last for several days. Keep refrigerated. In summer you can add organic fresh fruit: peaches, papaya, blueberries, strawberries, all berries, apricots, instead of banana. In winter, add apples, kiwi, oranges, tangelos, persimmons or pears, and if fresh is unavailable, try sugar-free, frozen organic fruits. Serves 1 to 2.

Patricia's Delicious Health Popcorn

Use freshly popped organic popcorn (use air popper). Drizzle organic olive oil, melted coconut oil or salt-free butter over popcorn. Sprinkle with good quality nutritional yeast for amazing flavor. For a variety try a pinch of cayenne pepper, mustard powder or fresh crushed garlic to oil mixture. Serve instead of breads!

Nutrition directly affects growth, development, reproduction, well-being of an individual's physical and mental condition. Health depends upon nutrition more than on any other single factor. – Dr. William H. Sebrell, Jr.

Lentil & Brown Rice Casserole, Burgers or Soup
Paul Bragg and Jack LaLanne's Favorite Recipe

16 oz pkg organic lentils, uncooked
1 cup brown organic rice, uncooked
5 cups, distilled / purified water
4-6 carrots, chop $^1/_2$" rounds
3 celery stalks, chop

4 garlic cloves, chop
2 onions, chop
2 tsps organic coconut aminos
1 tsp salt-free all-purpose seasoning
2 tsps organic extra-virgin olive oil

1 cup diced fresh or canned tomatoes (salt-free)

Wash and drain lentils and rice. Place grains in large stainless steel pot. Add water, bring to boil, reduce heat and simmer 30 minutes. Now add vegetables and seasonings and cook on low heat until tender. Last five minutes add fresh or canned (salt-free) tomatoes. For delicious garnish, add minced parsley & nutritional yeast. **For Burgers mash. For Soup, add more water in cooking grains.** Serves 4 to 6.

Raw Organic Vegetable Health Salad

2 stalks celery, chop
1 bell pepper & seeds, dice
$^1/_2$ cucumber, slice
2 carrots, grate
1 raw beet, grate
1 cup green cabbage, chop

$^1/_2$ cup red cabbage, chop
$^1/_2$ cup alfalfa, mung or sunflower sprouts
2 spring onions & green tops, chop
1 turnip, grate
1 avocado (ripe)
3 tomatoes, medium size

For variety add organic raw zucchini, peas, mushrooms, broccoli, cauliflower, (try black olives and pasta). Chop, slice or grate vegetables fine to medium for variety in size. Mix vegetables & serve on bed of lettuce, spinach, chopped kale or cabbage. Dice avocado and tomato and serve on side as a dressing. Serve choice of fresh squeezed lemon, orange or dressing separately. Chill salad plates before serving. **It's best to always eat salad first before hot dishes.** Serves 3 to 5.

131

Patricia's Health Salad Dressing

$^1/_2$ cup raw organic apple cider vinegar
1-2 tsps organic raw honey

$^1/_2$ tsp organic coconut aminos
1-2 cloves garlic, minced

$^1/_3$ cup organic extra-virgin olive oil, or blend with safflower, sesame or flax oil
1 Tbsp fresh herbs, minced (to taste)

Blend ingredients in blender or jar. Refrigerate in covered jar.

For delicious Herbal Vinegar: In quart jar add $^1/_3$ cup tightly packed, crushed fresh sweet basil, tarragon, dill, oregano, or any fresh herbs desired, combined or singly (if dried herbs, use 1-2 tsps herbs). Now cover to top with raw, organic apple cider vinegar and store two weeks in warm place, and then strain and refrigerate.

Honey – Chia or Celery Seed Vinaigrette

$^1/_4$ tsp dry mustard
$^1/_4$ tsp organic coconut aminos
$^1/_4$ tsp paprika or to taste
1-2 Tbsps honey

1 cup organic apple cider vinegar
$^1/_2$ cup organic extra-virgin olive oil
$^1/_2$ small onion, minced
$^1/_3$ tsp chia or celery seed (or vary to taste)

Blend ingredients in blender or jar. Refrigerate in covered jar.

Studies show both beta carotene and vitamin C, abundantly found in fruits and vegetables, play vital roles in preventing heart disease and cancers.

Fasting Cleanses, Renews and Rejuvenates

Our bodies have a natural self-cleansing method for maintaining a clean, healthy body and our "river of life" – our blood. It's essential we keep our entire bodily machinery from head to toes healthy and in good working order so nothing breaks down!

Fasting is the best detoxifying method. It's also the most effective and safest way to increase elimination of waste buildups and enhance the body's miraculous self-healing and self-repairing process that keeps you healthy and youthful.

If you prepare for a fast by eating a cleansing diet for 1 to 2 days, this can greatly facilitate the cleansing process. Fresh variety salads and organic vegetables, fruits and their juices, as well as green powder drinks (alfalfa, barley green, chlorella, spirulina, wheatgrass, etc.) stimulate waste elimination. Live, fresh foods and juices can literally pick up dead matter from your body and carry it away. After pre-cleansing period start your fast.

Daily, even on most fast days, we take from 1,000 to 3,000 mg. of mixed vitamin C powder *(try Emergen-C packs or C concentrate, acerola, rosehips, and bioflavonoid powders in liquids)*. This is a potent antioxidant and flushes out deadly free radicals. It also promotes collagen production for new healthy tissues. Also vitamin C and grapeseed extract are both important if you are detoxifying from prescription drugs or alcohol overload.

A peaceful, well planned distilled water fast is our favorite or the introductory fast of diluted fresh juice (with 35% distilled water). Both can cleanse your body of excess mucus, old fecal matter, trapped cellular, non-food wastes and help remove inorganic mineral deposits and sludge from your pipes and joints.

The miracle of fasting works by self-digestion. During a fast your body naturally will decompose and burn only the substances and tissues that are damaged, diseased or unneeded, such as abscesses, tumors, excess fat deposits, excess water and congestive wastes. Even a short fast (1-3 days) will accelerate

The nation badly needs to go on a diet. We should do something drastic about excessive, unattractive, life-threatening fat. We should get rid of harmful obesity in the quickest possible way and this is by fasting. – Allan Cott, M.D.

elimination from your liver, kidneys, lungs, bloodstream and skin. Sometimes you will experience dramatic changes (cleansing and healing crises) as accumulated wastes are expelled. With your first fasts you may temporarily have headaches, fatigue, body odor, bad breath, coated tongue, mouth sores and even diarrhea as your body is cleaning house. Please be patient with your body!

After a fast your body begins to healthfully rebalance when you faithfully follow The Bragg Healthy Lifestyle. Your weekly 24-hour fast removes toxins on a regular basis, so they don't accumulate. Your energy levels will rise and shine – physically, mentally, emotionally and spiritually. Your creativity expands. You will feel like a whole "new you" – which you are – you are being cleansed, purified and reborn. Fasting is a miracle!

Fasting – Is Master Key to Internal Purification

If you do a complete water fast for 24 hours each week, soon you will be able to add more fresh fruit and vegetables to your diet. We faithfully fast 24 hours every Monday and the first three days of each month. Wait until you experience this! You will greatly benefit from the inner cleansing – physically, mentally, emotionally and spiritually, and will love the pure, clean, healthy feeling you receive following this Bragg Healthy Lifestyle program!

133

Praises for Bragg Lifestyle & Miracle of Fasting

"Fasting is an effective and safe method of detoxifying the body . . . a technique that wise men have used for centuries to heal the sick. Fast regularly and help the body heal itself and stay well. Give all your organs a healthy rest. Fasting can help reverse the aging process, and if we use it correctly, we will live longer, happier lives. Just three days a month will do it. Each time you complete a fast, you will feel better. Your body will have a chance to heal and rebuild its immune system by regular fasting. You can fight off illness and the degenerative diseases so common in this chemically polluted environment we live in. When you feel a cold or any illness coming on or are just depressed – fast!"

– James Balch, M.D., co-author, *Prescription for Natural Healing*
"Bragg Books were my conversion to the healthy way."

(BENEFITS FROM THE JOYS OF FASTING)

Fasting renews your faith in yourself, your strength and God's strength.
Fasting is easier than any diet.
Fasting is the quickest way to lose weight.
Fasting is adaptable to a busy life.
Fasting gives the body a physiological rest.
Fasting is used successfully in the treatment of many physical illnesses.
Fasting can yield weight losses of up to 10 pounds or more in the first week.
Fasting lowers and normalizes cholesterol, homocysteine, blood pressure levels.
Fasting improves dietary habits.
Fasting increases pleasure eating healthy foods.
Fasting is a calming experience, often relieving tension and insomnia.
Fasting frequently induces feelings of happy euphoria, a natural high.
Fasting is a miracle rejuvenator, helps in slowing the ageing process.
Fasting is a natural stimulant to rejuvenate the growth hormone levels.
Fasting is an energizer, not a debilitator.
Fasting aids the elimination process.
Fasting often results in a more vigorous happy marital relationship.
Fasting can eliminate smoking, drug and drinking addictions.
Fasting is a regulator, educating the body to consume food only as needed.
Fasting saves precious time spent on marketing, preparing and eating.
Fasting rids the body of toxins, giving it an internal shower and cleansing.
Fasting does not deprive the body of essential nutrients.
Fasting can be used to uncover the sources of food allergies.
Fasting is used effectively in schizophrenia and other mental illness treatment.
Fasting under proper supervision can be tolerated easily up to four weeks.
Fasting does not accumulate appetite; hunger pangs disappear in 1-2 days.
Fasting is routine for most of the animal kingdom.
Fasting has been a common practice since the beginning of man's existence.
Fasting is practiced in all religions; the Bible alone has 74 references to fasting.
Fasting under proper conditions is absolutely safe.
Fasting is a blessing – "Fasting As A Way Of Life" – Allan Cott, M.D.
Fasting is not starving, it's nature's cure that God has given us. – Patricia Bragg

134

Dear Health Friend,

This gentle reminder explains the great benefits from "The Miracle of Fasting" that you will enjoy when starting on your weekly 24-hour Bragg Fasting Program for Super Health! It's a precious time of body-mind-soul cleansing and renewal.

On fast days I drink 8-10 glasses of distilled (our favorite) or purified water, (I add 1-2 tsps. organic, raw apple cider vinegar to three of them). If just starting, you may also try herbal teas or try diluted fresh juices with 1/3 distilled water. Every day, even on fast days, add 1 Tbsp. of psyllium husk powder to liquids once daily. It's an extra cleanser and helps normalize weight, cholesterol and blood pressure and helps promote healthy elimination. Fasting is the oldest, most effective healing method known to man. Fasting offers great miraculous blessings from Mother Nature and our Creator. It begins the self-cleansing of the inner-body workings so we can promote our own self-healing.

My father and I wrote the book "The Miracle of Fasting" to share with you the health miracles it can perform in your life. It's all so worthwhile to do. It's an important part of The Bragg Healthy Lifestyle.

With Love, Patricia

Paul Bragg's work on fasting and water is one of the great contributions to The Healing Wisdom and The Natural Health Movement in the world today.
– Gabriel Cousens, M.D., Author "Conscious Eating" and "Spiritual Nutrition"

Chapter 9

We Need Pure Water for Health

Drink Only Healthy, Pure Distilled Water

Other than fruit and vegetable juices, my father and I would drink no other liquid except steam-produced distilled water. Today, in this polluted and poisoned world, distilled water is the purest water on the face of the earth. It contains no solid matter of any kind. It is made solely of two elements, hydrogen and oxygen. There are no minerals in it, organic or inorganic. It can be used as drinking water and cooking water and also can be used in electric steam irons.

When distilled water enters the body, it leaves no residue of any kind. It's free of salt and sodium. It's also the most perfect water to promote healthy functioning of those great "sieves," the kidneys. It's the perfect liquid for the blood. It's the ideal liquid for efficient functioning of the lungs, stomach, liver and all of your vital organs.

135

Why? Because it's free of all inorganic minerals! It's essential for the formulation of liquid drug prescriptions. Also, it's important for kidney and heart patients.

Let no person tell you that distilled water is dead water! Of course, fish will not live in distilled water. Fish require vegetation growth, seaweed, etc. in water and vegetable growth needs inorganic minerals to live.

What is "Pure Water"?

Reading this book, *Water – The Shocking Truth,* you are becoming aware of the pros and cons of distilled water versus mineral or ground water. Unfortunately, however, writers and lecturers are now creating confusion about distilled water. Some have actually referred to "soft water" (water treated by a water softener) as "distilled water." This is definitely not the case! Softened water has a high content of inorganic sodium, calcium and other inorganic minerals.

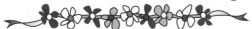

We all grow healthier in nature, gentle sunshine, pure water and love!

Using this misinformation as a basis, even some health publications have made misleading comparisons in an attempt to make a case against distilled water! For example, group comparisons were made citing people who lived in remote areas with hard ground water supplies and yet had a low incidence of cardiovascular (heart and circulatory system) problems – without also taking into consideration the pertinent fact that such people tend to eat more natural "live" foods and live in a relaxed, rural environment!

On the basis of water alone, this rural group was compared with people living in crowded, highly polluted metropolitan areas who drank treated city water, presumably filtered through home water softeners (erroneously designated as "distilled water"), who also showed a higher incidence of hypertension and other cardiovascular problems. No mention was made of the obvious facts that these urban dwellers were subjected to much greater tensions, as well as diets of lifeless, processed "plastic" foods from supermarket shelves – both major contributors to cardiovascular illnesses.

136

Obviously, any self-styled "researcher" who makes such errors as those noted above has not done their basic homework! Unfortunately, the reader may not be aware of this – and thus unnecessary confusion is irresponsibly created. So, with water as with eating, don't let the so-called "experts," often paid by big interest violators, fool you!

What is Distilled Water? The Best for Health!

Throughout this book we have stressed that distilled water is the only pure water – the only water you should put into your body. As noted previously, "soft water" is not distilled water . . . nor is "purified water," "deionized water," "filtered water" or "reverse osmosis water."

There is only one process that can make 100% distilled water and that is steam distillation. In steam distillation, only pure water (H_2O) evaporates, leaving all inorganic minerals and other impurities behind.

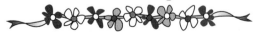

The best method for purifying your water is a system that distills your water and then carbon filters it. – Dr. Robert Willix, Jr.

What About Rain Water?

Rain water once was the ideal distilled water. Today, in some areas, air has toxic pollution that contaminates and poisons this natural water.

Toxins such as Strontium 90 from beacons to bombs and the exhaust from airplanes and automobiles turn rain water into a deadly poison. Vicious toxins are sent into the air from our industrial factories – sulfur dioxides, lead, carbon monoxide and hundreds of pollutants.

So, in our present civilization, drinking rain water in some areas is not advised! To live in this poisoned world, to survive and save ourselves from other kinds of destruction (the complete solidification of the body, brain structures, etc.), please drink only distilled water!

Pure Water Fights Hardening of the Arteries

We do not want our brain, arteries and other blood vessels to turn into stone! You see this condition every day in prematurely old people suffering from dementia. Often you hear the word "fossil" used to describe the prehistoric remnants of animals who lived on earth ages ago. When you drink a glass of ordinary tap water, the process of fossilization has already begun.

Many times we've heard someone say something such as, "That old fossil John Smith died last night from hardening of the arteries." Although the remark was crude, it was truthful! If we escape the other deadly degenerative and infectious diseases in this life, we are still haunted by that silent deadly killer of mankind worldwide, "hardening of the arteries."

Rainwater is not as pure as you might expect. Despite sometimes aggressive marketing claims, drinking rainwater has not been shown to be more beneficial than other sources of clean drinking water. It is prudent to never assume that rainwater is safe to drink. Rain can wash different types of contaminants into the water you collect. – waterandhealth.org

Be determined that you are going to drink only pure distilled water. If you cannot get it delivered from a water company, try health or grocery stores. Also, most drug stores carry distilled water for people with heart and kidney problems. Don't wait until these happen to you!

If you cannot find distilled water for sale, purchase a small water distiller and make your own pure water. You may say it's a lot of trouble – but it's not nearly as much trouble as when your arteries harden and your body is slowly starved for want of oxygen and health!

Remember, the bloodstream carries vital oxygen to all parts of the body. Also if arteries become encrusted with inorganic minerals, you are in for grave problems. Oxygen starvation causes a host of serious ailments.

Stages of Artery Hardening

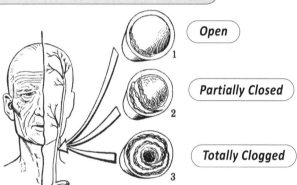

This drawing shows the 3 stages of the hardening of blood vessels in the brain. As the flow of blood becomes slower, clots may form and completely close a vessel.

Open

Partially Closed

Totally Clogged

138

We Drink Juices During Our World Health Crusades

At times we were unable to find distilled water during our many Bragg Health Crusades which carried us around the world. But when it wasn't available – or if we were in doubt about the water supply – for short periods we let fresh raw vegetables, fruits and their juices supply us with their naturally pure water. We always had a small hand citrus juicer with us for our fresh orange or grapefruit juice. Fresh and organic is always best for your health!

There is only one water that is clean and that is steam distilled water. No other substance on our planet does so much to keep us healthy and get us well as this water does. – Dr. James Balch, author of "Rx Prescription for Dietary Wellness"

Man is as old as his arteries. – Rudolf Virchow, 1821-1902 German Doctor, Father of Pathology and Social Medicine

Man is as Old as His Arteries

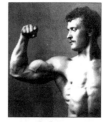

"Father of Modern Body Building," Eugen Sandow's athletic strength and prowess didn't save him from having a massive coronary. He died at 58! The autopsy showed that his arteries were like stone.

Eugen Sandow, greatest strong man of all times, was a friend of Dads. When he visited him in his studio in London, he would flex his muscles and say how powerful he was. But he drank London tap water and at 58 he had a massive coronary. His great strength and bulging muscles could not save his life. There is absolutely no way to circumvent this powerful truth. Another example was demonstrated during the Korean War, when autopsies were performed on 300 young American soldiers that were killed within a short period. What do you think was revealed? Shockingly – all of these young men showed signs of hardening of the arteries! This scientific study is on record. These were young men under 23, in the so-called prime of life, suffering from degeneration (fossilizing) of the body's arteries.

Life Expectancy – Life Span

We are told that a male child born today has a life expectancy of 75-78 years, and a female child 80-83. What is the actual life span of the average American?

We can surmise that when a male reaches 37 years he has lived about half of his lifetime, and when a female reaches 40 years she has lived about half of her lifetime. The sad but true fact is that some people never even reach their expected life span. See website: *worldbank.org/data*

The U.S. and countries around the globe are experiencing epidemics of heart disease and cancer. Consider this startling fact: chances are better than 2 to 1 that, the average American adult will die of some form of heart disease or cancer. You as an individual can reverse this shocking statistic by avoiding ordinary water that is laced with inorganic minerals and toxins. Start drinking only distilled water today (*8 glasses daily*).

The oldest confirmed recorded age for any human is 122 years – a lady in France.

Exercise is Vital for Youthful Arteries

For youthful arteries, exercise is essential! If you wish to live a long, healthy life it is necessary to build up your cardiovascular endurance and to follow a program designed to keep your arteries soft and agile.

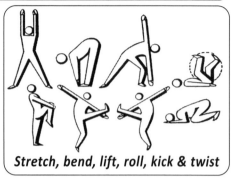

Stretch, bend, lift, roll, kick & twist

The first step is to get more oxygen into the body which will help dissolve the encrustations that have formed in the arteries. Any physical activity that injects more oxygen is going to help extend your life! Get out and jog, swim, ride a bike or take a brisk 2 to 3 mile energizing walk.

The Great Watermelon Flush

140

There is nothing like a watermelon flush to dissolve and eliminate inorganic minerals from your entire body.

As a youth, my father had a history of drinking exceptionally hard water loaded with inorganic minerals. The contaminants in that hard water encrusted the pipes of his body, and when he learned the truth of the great damage it could do to his system, he started to experiment with fruits and vegetables to find out which one had the greatest encrustation-dissolving power. It was a long search, but at last he found watermelon and its juice to provide the cleansing miracle.

Several times a year we went on a watermelon flush by eating nothing for 5 to 7 days but watermelon and watermelon juice. Every morning we took a sample of the very first urine we voided. We would seal it tightly, date it and put it on a shelf for 6 months to a year. As it broke down, the inorganic minerals, which are heavier, settle on the bottom of the bottle. Having studied biochemistry, my father analyzed the substances and found calcium carbonate, magnesium carbonate and many other inorganic minerals, chemicals and toxins.

Studies have shown that brisk walking just 15 minutes or more a day helps maintain healthy blood vessels for good circulation in the body and brain.

That is why we went on a watermelon flush several times a year and often would make it our lunch meal. It's best not to mix melons with other foods. We also eat watermelon during its season. On an average day in the hot summertime, we will drink as much as 1 to 2 quarts of watermelon juice.

Prevention is Always Better than a Cure

Although most people seldom realize it, they live continually under the fear of sickness and death. They would even indignantly deny this assertion and insist they are not afraid to die – although most of us are willing to admit the fear of developing some deadly disease or physical condition that may make us a less efficient human than we are now.

People always fear the unknown: for that very reason we have learned to expect catastrophes from many unanticipated sources. But if we fully understand what disease is, how it originates and become familiar with the only avenues through which illness can strike us, then what have we to fear except ourselves?

To prevent disease is to circumvent the daily cause of illness . . . which, as previously discussed, is the clogging of our bodies with deadly chemicals and inorganic minerals, salt and the increasing amounts of toxic, acid by-products of digestion and metabolism – all conditions which we can control by our lifestyle.

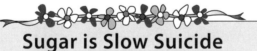

Sugar is Slow Suicide

High sugar consumption can overstimulate and harm your whole body system. Research Studies revealed one of the biggest hidden threats to health is consumption of fructose, sucrose, and all other forms of sugar, which can lead to many serious health problems, ranging from: obesity, cancer, and heart trouble, to high blood sugar levels and diabetes. – *Dr. David Williams, "Mayo Clinic Guide to Healthy Living"*

 Whatsoever was the father of a disease; an ill diet was the mother. – George Herbert

So, if we can recover from disease by a reversal of our wrong habits of living, won't these same good habits prevent disease in the first place? Prevention may cost little, but it sure saves a lot! If one is of sound mind, it must seem clear that the only sane method is to avoid an unhealthy lifestyle that causes disease. Prevention is the best way to feel and remain youthful, energetic and virile throughout a long, healthy, fulfilled life.

If we are to prevent disease, we must have a basic rudimentary knowledge of our bodies. Our bodies are composed of millions of cells bathed in an electrolytic solution consisting of organic calcium, magnesium, potassium, sodium and phosphorus, with trace amounts of copper and zinc. These are all organic minerals (see page 87). The body cannot use inorganic minerals for building its cells. These electrolytes are held in solution by water, which makes up 75% of the body. For this reason, we can live without food for long periods, but we can only live about 72 hours without water. So you can see how important it is that the body not only get sufficient water, but the right kind of water. Distilled water is important for super health and longevity!

The vast majority of people drink ordinary tap water laced with chemicals and inorganic minerals. Your body can make no selections for itself, but must accept what you put into it. When you give your body water that is heavily loaded with chemicals and inorganic minerals, your body has to do something with these poisons. It therefore stores them in your arteries, veins, joints, eyes, ears, nose, throat, gallbladder and other vital organs.

Our Bodies Can Only Endure So Much Severe Punishment and Still Survive!

Because the body is such a miracle instrument, it can take a great deal of punishment and still function. For many years the body seems to handle the situation. But the day finally arrives when the poisons you have loaded into your body begin to give you trouble – real trouble: increasing pain, suffering, misery and agony!

_____

The power of pure water is the vital chemistry of life!

Those people who have laughed in Mother Nature's face now cry out in pain, "Help me! Save me from my terrible suffering!" These are the people who want a cure. A cure? No one can cure you of anything!

Only the basic biological functions of the body can perform a cure. Don't wait until pain strikes to start taking care of your wonderful body! It may be too late then. Today is the day to outline a healthy lifestyle program for yourself and live by it faithfully hereafter. You get only one body during your lifetime. If you want to live in health and freedom from suffering, you must faithfully follow the Health Laws of Mother Nature. These are good laws. They support you having a painless, tireless, ageless body. It's your birthright to feel the thrill of joyous living every day of your entire life!

By following Mother Nature's laws you can awaken one beautiful morning to discover the feeling of radiant health and happiness! You'll have slept deeply like a baby. Gone are your headaches, gone is your chronic fatigue, gone are all your aches and pains! You'll feel new vitality surging throughout your entire body. You'll have a spring in your step, a sparkle in your eyes and the glow of health in your skin. You'll have found the greatest and most precious treasure in the whole world – radiant, glorious health! Physical and mental health are now yours!

143

Perpetual Youthfulness Can Be Yours!

Longfellow said that, "In youth the heart exults and sings!" This suggests the idea that beyond certain prescribed years that the heart does not exult and sing. Youth, in its crudest sense, does not refer to years but to a state of being. It really is a matter of one's own choice, if one is born with a normal constitution, as to when youth shall end and "middle age" begin. Some people can truly be referred to as youthful although they may have seen sixty or more years.

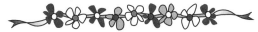

To preserve health is a moral and religious duty, for health is the basis for all social virtues. We can't be as useful when not well.
– Dr. Samuel Johnson, Father of Dictionaries, 1709-1784

Most people have a desire to remain youthful, but few are willing to pay the price. The price of prolonged youthfulness is the consistent faithful performance of certain healthy lifestyle habits. These healthy lifestyle habits are: staying away from chemicalized drinking water full of inorganic minerals; eating no salt; drinking ample amounts of distilled water; eating a healthy, well-balanced, natural diet; consistent daily exercise; deep power breathing; good personal hygiene; and thinking positively! Without a healthy body, it is difficult to maintain positive thinking!

You now know that the most destructive force that robs you of youthful good health consists of a gradual settling of insoluble inorganic mineral matter from water and salt into the tissues of your body. This encrustation begins first on the walls of the arteries, gradually diminishing their elasticity and caliber as well as the nourishment of the tissues they supply.

As a consequence of these destructive changes, all body functions slow down more and more until some vital organ then stops altogether and death occurs from premature ageing. The beginning of corrosion and the subsequent hardening of the arteries are the first stages of premature ageing, no matter how long a person has lived!

Your life-long work is the battle to keep your arteries free from the inorganic minerals and toxic chemicals contained in most drinking water. Stop using table salt and eat a balanced diet that does not leave a residue of toxic crystals to clog and obstruct your circulation.

You now know what we know . . . the shocking truth about water . . . and what we believe to be the world's best-kept health secret. Let's really make life a healthful, vigorous adventure! Health and happiness are our goals. Health is our wealth! There is success ahead for those who start today and faithfully move steadily onward in their quest for radiant, youthful health!

The great thing in life is not so much where you stand, but in what direction you are moving – right (positive) or wrong (negative).

I have found perfect health, a new state of existence, a feeling of purity and happiness, something unknown to humans!
– Novelist Upton Sinclair, a frequent faster

Paul C. Bragg's Prediction

Mine is only a small voice in the vast wilderness concerning this matter of drinking only distilled water, but I sincerely wish to save humanity from the dangers of water filled with chemicals and inorganic minerals.

I have lived a long life. During this time I have seen some of my relatives and personal friends, as well as some 200 animals and friends' pets die of fossilization.

I believe I am a hundred years ahead of my time in my theories on the dangers of inorganic water and an unhealthy lifestyle. Someday humanity will recognize the dangers in ordinary water and all water used in homes, schools, hospitals, etc. will be steam distilled! It will be the greatest health advancement this world has ever known!

No matter how much a person controls his eating habits . . . no matter how much juice of organic fruits and vegetables he drinks, no matter if he lives on a raw food, vegetarian or so-called modern scientific diet . . . as long as he continues to drink spring, well, river, lake or fluoridated and chlorinated water he is going to fossilize himself! In the past 75 years I have met all the greats in the fields of nutrition, natural healing, etc., but most of them drank the water filled with chemicals and inorganic mineral water, unaware of the dangers and only a few of them attained a long, pain free, healthy life.

The same is true of the great athletes of the past 75 years. They had their day in the sun, drank the deadly inorganic mineral water and died at about the same age as non-athletic people.

I was personally acquainted with Bill Tilden, the greatest tennis player of all time. In his prime, no man in the world could defeat him. But he would not listen to my lone, small voice when I told him of the viciousness and deadliness of inorganic mineral water. He said that everybody else was drinking ordinary water, so he saw no reason he should stop. He died at age 60 from coronary thrombosis. (Read next page for facts on why distilled water is best for your health).

21 FACTS ABOUT DISTILLED WATER

You should know that Distilled Water . . .

- is water that's been turned into vapor so that its impurities are left behind. Upon condensing, it becomes pure distilled water.
- is the only type of water that meets the definition of water: hydrogen + oxygen.
- is a perfectly natural healthy water.
- is also odorless, colorless and tasteless.
- is free of virtually all inorganic minerals, including salt.
- is the only natural solvent that can be taken into the body without damage to the tissues.
- acts as a solvent in the body by dissolving nutrients so they can be assimilated and taken into every cell.
- dissolves the cell wastes so the toxins can be removed.
- dissolves inorganic mineral substances lodged in the tissues of the body so that such substances can be eliminated in the process of purifying the body.

- does not leach out organic body minerals but collects and removes the toxic inorganic minerals which have been rejected by the cells and are therefore nothing more than harmful debris obstructing the normal functions of the body.
- is indeed the most ideal and beneficial water for all humans and also for animals.
- leaves no residue of any kind when it enters the body.
- is the most perfect water for the healthy functioning of those great miracle sieves, the kidneys.
- is the perfect liquid for the blood.
- is the ideal liquid for efficient functioning of the lungs, stomach, liver and all other vital organs.
- is universally accepted as the standard for biomedical applications and for drinking water purity.
- is so pure that all drug prescriptions are formulated with distilled water.
- is fresh, clean and pleasing to the palate.
- makes foods and drinks prepared with it taste noticeably better. The flavor is subtle enough not to interfere with the food it is mixed with.
- is the only pure water left on our polluted planet!
- Remember – Distilled Water is the healthiest water and the greatest natural water on earth!

Chapter 10

Water Used in Your Home

Tap Water – Danger in Every Glass

Water from chemically-treated public water systems – and even from many wells and springs – is likely to be loaded with poisonous chemicals and toxic trace elements! Depending upon the kind of piping that the water has been run through, the water in our homes, offices, schools, hospitals, etc., is likely to be overloaded with zinc (from old-fashioned galvanized pipes) or with copper and cadmium (from copper pipes). These trace elements are released in large quantities by the chemical action of the water on the metals of the pipes.

Filtered Distilled Tap Water – Best for Health

The best method of ensuring a safe water supply in your home is to install a home water distillation system. It's the only purification system that removes every kind of bacteria, virus, parasite, and pathogen, as well as pesticides, herbicides, organic and inorganic chemicals, heavy metals and even radioactive contaminants. In a properly made distillation system, tap water is preheated to just below boiling point to drive off compounds that are lighter than water (volatile organic compounds or VOCs). Once those compounds have evaporated, water is heated just to boiling point then sent to a condensation chamber to return to its liquid state as pure, distilled water.

147

A filtration system, and changing filters often, can purify your tap water, but, as with bottled water, filtration systems must be evaluated and consumer lab reports given careful study. Some systems remove up to 99% of THMs (trihalomethane toxic chemical by-product when chlorine is used to disinfect drinking water) and synthetic organic compounds. All less efficient systems provide a false sense of security to consumers. (Filtered water is NOT distilled water.) We've researched the processes and equipment available for making distilled water. We encourage you to review new equipment as it comes on the market too. Please see the water system comparison chart on next page.

Comparison of Water Treatment Methods Show Steam Distilled Water is the Best

Pollutant	Sediment Filter	Carbon Filter	Reverse Osmosis	Steam Distillation
Aluminum	○	○	●	●
Arsenic	○	○	◐	●
Bacteria	○	○	◐	●
Benzene	○	○	●[1]	●[1]
Bromide	○	○	●	●
Cadmium	○	○	●	●
Calcium	○	○	●	●
Chlorides	○	●	●	●
Chlorine	○	●	●[1]	●[1]
Chromium (VI)	○	◐	●[1]	●[1]
Cryptosporidium	○	○	●	●
Detergents	○	◐	●	●
Fluorides	○	○	●	●
Herbicides	○	●	●[1]	●[1]
Lead	○	○	●	●
Magnesium	○	○	●	●
Mercury	○	○	●	●
MTBE	○	●	●[1]	●[1]
Nitrate	○	○	◐	●
Organics	○	●	●[1]	●[1]
Pesticides	○	●	●[1]	●[1]
Phosphates	○	○	●	●
Radon	○	○	●[1]	●[1]
Sediment	●	◐	●	●
Sodium	○	○	●	●
Sulfates	○	◐	●	●
Sulfide	○	◐	●	●
TDS	○	○	●	●
TTHM	○	○	●[1]	●[1]
Viruses	○	○	○	●

○ Ineffective or No Reduction   ◐ Significant Reduction   ● Effective Removal

1 – A Carbon Filter Needed (The best home distillers also have carbon filters.)

The kind of water you drink can make or break you – your body is 75% water.

Nature's Health Tonic is Distilled Water . . .

**It's free of all inorganic minerals and toxic chemicals.
You will enjoy it's many benefits from drinking it:**

- Water regulates all body functions. It is essential for the removal of wastes, especially from body tissues.
- Water keeps skin from dehydrating and wrinkling; leaving it healthy, resilient, looking years younger.
- Water helps to maintain a healthier muscle tone.
- Distilled water will help you lose weight. It helps suppress any unhealthy over-eating, stuffing habits and suppresses the appetite naturally!
- Drinking lots of distilled water is the best treatment for fluid retention, for it helps remove body toxins.
- Daily 8-10 glasses of distilled water helps banish constipation and aids the body to eliminate waste more regularly.

Yes – drinking 8-10 glasses distilled water daily is the master key to health and vigor! It's preventative to help protect us from this poisonous industrial age! It's a vital fluid that helps keep our bodies healthy!

Distilled Water Acts as a Natural Cleansing Solvent in the Body

The purer water is (free from inorganic minerals, dissolved heavy metals, softeners, pollutants, etc.) the more toxins it can absorb and carry out of the body; also, the more nutrients it will be able to carry to the body's cells. Other fluids made from water like coffee, alcohol, tea, cola drinks, etc. are already saturated with pollutants and are less able to absorb and carry away toxins. Incredible as it may seem, water is quite possibly the single most important catalyst in losing weight and keeping it off! Although most of us take it for granted, water may be the only true 'magic potion' for permanent weight loss! It's usually best not to drink beverages with meals, as it dilutes the digestive enzymes! Drink water up to $1/2$ hour before or not less than $1/2$ hour after meals.

*There is no trifling with nature; it is always true, dignified, and just;
it is always in the right, and the faults and errors belong to us.
Nature defies incompetence, but reveals its secrets to the competent,
the truthful, and the pure. – Johann Wolfgang von Goethe*

Clean & Detoxify with Pure Distilled Water

Each healthy individual body requires a proper balance within itself of all the nutritive elements. It is just as bad for an individual to have too much of one item as it is to have too little of another one. It takes appropriate levels of phosphorus and magnesium to keep calcium in solution so that it can be transformed into new cells of bone and teeth. Yet, there must not be too much of those nutrients, nor too little calcium in the diet, or old bone will be taken away, but new bone will not be formed. Additionally, we now know that diets which are unbalanced and inappropriate for a given individual can deplete the body of calcium, magnesium, potassium and other major and minor elements.

Diets which are high in meats, fish, eggs, and refined grains and their products may provide unbalanced excesses of phosphorus which will deplete calcium and magnesium from the bones and tissues of the body, causing those minerals to be lost in the urine. A diet high in fats will tend to increase the intake of phosphorus from the intestines relative to calcium and other basic minerals. Such a high-fat diet can result in the loss of calcium, magnesium and other basic nutrients in much the same way a high-phosphorus diet does.

Diets excessively high in fruits or their juices may provide unbalanced excesses of sugar and potassium in the body, and calcium and magnesium will again be lost from the body through urine. These calcium and magnesium deficiencies can produce many problems in the body, ranging from dental decay, diabetes and osteoporosis to muscular cramping and twitching, hyperactivity, poor sleep patterns, and excessive frequency and uncontrolled urination. Similarly, deficiencies of other minerals or imbalances can produce other problems.

Lack of water is the #1 trigger of daytime fatigue!

Let food be your medicine, and medicine be your food. – Hippocrates

Enjoy healthy, organic foods for their wonderful abundance of life energy.

One solution to America's soaring health costs is pure distilled water.

Despite numerous dietary sources such as these, many adults and children in so-called civilized cultures will be found to have low levels of essential minerals in their bodies due to losses caused by drinking coffee, tea, and carbonated beverages, combined with the long-term habit of eating bad, "plastic" foods containing too much sugar and table salt, as well as products made from refined flours! In addition, the body's organs can be thrown out of balance by continued stress, toxins in our air and water, along with disease-produced injuries or pre-natal deficiencies linked to the mother's unhealthy diet or lifestyle! As a result, many if not most people in our so-called civilization may need to take a natural chelated multiple mineral supplement as well as a broad-range multiple vitamin for extra insurance.

Therefore, it's important to clean and detoxify your body through fasting and drinking pure distilled water and moderate amounts of organically-grown vegetable and fruit juices. It's also important to provide the body with an adequate source of new minerals. This can be done by eating a variety of healthy organic vegetables, including kelp and other sea vegetables for adults and natural healthy mother's milk for infants.

Human Cell is Immortal Says Dr. Alexis Carrel

Dr. Alexis Carrel, pioneer scientist at the Rockefeller Institute, won the greatest award, the Nobel Prize in Medicine by demonstrating his arresting hypotheses: "The Cell is Immortal". It's merely the fluid in which it floats that degenerates. Renew fluid at regular intervals, give the cells what they require and as far as we know, the pulsation of life may go on forever. His hypotheses was that, premature death and many symptoms of the body's ageing process are due to accumulation of toxins in the body cells. These toxins are from cellular decay and also enter your body in the air you breathe, food you eat and water you drink. This overload of toxins keeps your body from absorbing and utilizing nutrition your cells so desperately need. According to Dr. Carrel, if your cells are cleansed of all toxins and proper nutrients are provided, you should be able to live without ageing!

Since your body is 75% water, the blood and lymphatic system is over 90% water, it's essential for your health that you consistently drink only pure distilled water that's not saturated with contaminants, inorganic minerals and toxins! This water helps transport vital nutrients to cells and waste from cells more efficiently. This allows the body to function correctly and stay healthier! See Dr. Alexis Carrel on web: www.nobelprize.org

Don't Drink Dangerous, Toxic Fluoride!

Fluoride is among the most potentially dangerous of all water additives! Long-term research into fluoridation has shown that its positive effects on dental health are minimal at best (page 29) and are far outweighed by the serious health risks (page 32) resulting from its use. Cancer researcher Dr. Dean Burke believes that 10% of all cancer deaths in the U.S. may be due directly to fluoridation! Yet, 80% of the citizenry continue drinking fluoridated water. Dr. Burke and associate, pioneer Dr. John Yiamouyiannis, both concluded drinking fluoridated water increases ones risk of cancer (see recommended reading page 173-176).

Fluoride has a voracious appetite for enzymes needed for healthy digestion, thereby reducing your body's ability to absorb vitamins essential for good health. While the fluoride debate continues, some authorities believe fluoride may cause birth defects, genetic damage, cancer and allergic responses. More immediately apparent is dental fluorosis, a gross mottling of young people's teeth (page 29), damage to the skeletal system (pages 30-31) and thyroid function (page 32). Former Auckland Principal Dental Officer, Dr. John Colquhoun, was an instigator of fluoridation in New Zealand. However, after much research, seeing toxic long-term effects of fluoride consumption, Dr. John Colquhoun became one of the foremost opponents of fluoridation! For more info on fluoride dangers reread pages 21-37.

How Safe is Chlorinated Water?

An estimated 98% of drinking water in the U.S. is chlorinated. While chlorination has helped to reduce the incidence of infectious diseases, known carcinogens such as chloroform and other trihalomethanes are formed when chlorine reacts with organic compounds in the water. These chemical compounds accumulate in fatty tissue such as breast tissues and can be found in body fat, blood, mothers' milk and even semen. Studies have implicated chlorinated drinking water with colorectal and bladder cancers! Highly chlorinated water resulted in a noticeable shift in the transformation of cholesterol from beneficial HDL to harmful LDL (pages 52-55).

The *American Journal of Public Health* published the results of a study of cancer risk over an 8 year period in 28,237 postmenopausal women. Those who drank water from municipal surface water sources consumed higher levels of chloroform than those who drank municipal ground water sources. The higher intake of chloroform was associated with an increased risk of colon cancer, and of all cancers combined.

Even chlorination does not provide full protection against the deadliest organisms in public water supplies. Cryptosporidium, a toxic parasitic protozoan, is chlorine resistant and is inadequately removed by sand filters.

"The worldwide pollution of lakes, streams, rivers and oceans and the chlorination of swimming pool water has led to an increase in deadly melanoma cancer."

– Reports Franz Rampen in *Epidemiology*

Skin Absorbs Water, Toxins and All*

(*from the *American Journal of Public Health*)

153

Compared with its absorption through the respiratory system, skin absorption could be the major route of penetration into the body! Skin penetration rates have been found to be remarkably high, and the outer layer of skin is a less effective barrier to penetration than traditionally assumed. Factors affecting absorption are:

HYDRATION: The more hydrated the skin, the greater the absorption. If the skin is hydrated (through perspiration or immersion in water) or if the contaminant compounds are in solution, diffusion and penetration will be enhanced.

TEMPERATURE: Increased skin or water temperature will enhance the skins absorption capacity proportionately. During swimming and bathing, it then demonstrates that greater hydration of skin surfaces will take place.

SKIN CONDITION: Any insult (i.e. sunburn) or injury (i.e. cuts, wounds, abrasions) to the skin will lower its ability to act as a barrier against foreign substances! A history of skin disease such as psoriasis or eczema acts to lower the natural barrier of the outer skin layer, as do rashes, dermatitis, or any chronic skin condition.

More men fail through lack of purpose, than lack of talent. – Billy Sunday

REGIONAL VARIABILITY: Skin absorption rates vary with different regions of the body. Underestimated is the case of whole body immersion during swimming or bathing. The epidermis of the hand represents a relatively greater barrier of penetration than many other parts of the body, including the scalp, forehead, abdomen, area in and around the ears, underarms and genital area. Penetration through the genital area is estimated to be 100%, but only 8.6% for the forearm.

OTHER ROUTES OF ENTRY: Other significant routes of absorption include through the oral, nasal, and mouth cavities, and eye and ear areas. These routes have been underestimated in their ability to absorb contaminants during immersion in water. Inhalation serves another route. In swimming or bathing, the volatilized chemicals are likely to gather near water surface and then are more readily inhalable. In addition, some water may be swallowed in these situations. *(During the 1984 Olympics in Los Angeles, the West German Swimming Team refused to compete in Olympic pool until chlorine was removed and an alternate purification method was installed.)*

154

More Toxins Are Absorbed From Taking A Shower Than From Drinking the Same Water!*

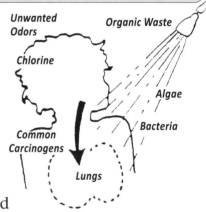

Two highly volatile and toxic chemicals, trichloroethylene (THMs) and chloroform have been proven as toxic contaminants found in most municipal drinking-water supplies. The National Academy of Sciences has estimated that hundreds of people die in the United States each year from cancers caused largely by ingesting water pollutants from inhalation as air pollutants in the home. Inhalation exposure to water pollutants is largely ignored. Data indicates that hot showers can liberate about 50% of the chloroform and 80% of the trichloroethylene into the air.

*from "Science News Magazine" • www.ScienceNews.org

Tests show that your body can absorb more toxic chlorine as a result of a 10-minute shower than if you drank 8 glasses of the same water. How can that be?

A warm shower opens up your pores, causing your skin to act like a sponge. As a result, you not only inhale the chlorine vapors, you absorb them through your skin, directly into your bloodstream – at a rate that's up to 6 times higher than if you were directly drinking it.

In terms of cumulative damage to your health, showering in chlorinated water is one of the most dangerous risks you take daily! Short-term risks include: eye, sinus, throat, skin and lung irritation. Long-term risks include: excessive free radial formation (that ages you!), higher vulnerability to genetic mutation and cancer development, and difficulty metabolizing cholesterol which can cause hardened arteries (*ScienceNews.com*).

Five Hidden Dangers in Your Shower:

- **Chlorine:** Added to all municipal water supplies, this disinfectant hardens arteries, destroys proteins in the body, irritates skin and sinus conditions and aggravates any asthma, allergy and respiratory problems.
- **Chloroform:** This powerful by-product of chlorination causes excessive free radical formation (accelerated ageing!), normal cells to mutate and cholesterol to form. Chlorine is a known carcinogen! Guard and protect your precious body.
- **DCA (Dichloroacetic acid):** This chlorine by-product alters the cholesterol metabolism and has been shown to cause health issues and liver cancer in lab animals.
- **MX (another chlorinated acid):** Another by-product of chlorination, MX is known to cause genetic mutations (induces DNA damage) that can lead to cancer growth and has been found in all chlorinated water for which it was tested.
- **Proven cause of bladder and rectal cancer:** Research proved that chlorinated water is the direct cause of 9% of all U.S. bladder cancers and 15% of all rectal cancers.

You can save yourself much money and the anxiety of falling ill by paying attention to your body's constant need for pure water.
– Dr. F. Batmanghelidj, author "Your Body's Many Cries For Water"

What Experts Have To Say About Showers, Toxic Chemicals & Chlorine

Water chlorination has been widely used to "purify" water in America starting in 1904. But chlorine's negative effects on health surely outweigh any benefits! "Chlorine is the greatest crippler and killer of modern times! While it prevented epidemics of one disease, it was creating another. Twenty years after the start of chlorinating our drinking water, the present mounting epidemic of heart trouble, cancer and senility began in 1924, and is costing billions." – Dr. Joseph M. Price, author of *Coronaries, Cholesterol, Chlorine*

Skin absorption of toxic dangerous contaminants has been greatly underestimated and the ingestion may not constitute the sole primary route of exposure. – Dr. Halina Brown, *American Journal of Public Health*

156

Taking long hot showers is a health risk, according to the latest research. Showers – and to a lesser extent baths – lead to a greater exposure to toxic chemicals contained in water supplies than does drinking the water. These toxic chemicals evaporate out of the water and are inhaled. They can also spread through the house and be inhaled by others. People get six to 100 times more chemicals by breathing the air while taking showers and baths than they would by drinking the water. – Ian Anderson, *New Scientist*

A Professor of Water Chemistry at the University of Pittsburgh claims that exposure to vaporized chemicals in the water through showering, bathing and inhalation is 100 times greater than through drinking the chemicals in water. – *The Nader Report – Troubled Waters on Tap*

Chlorination of the U.S. water supply is sufficient reason not to drink and shower in it – only use distilled water. – Marilyn Diamond, co-author of *Fit for Life*

To help retard the processes of premature and decrepit old age, it is essential that you drink plenty of distilled water daily. – Dr. Norman W. Walker, author of *Water Can Undermine Your Health*

Steam distillation is an extremely effective method of guarding against waterborne mirco-organisms because such contaminants cannot vaporize.

Don't Gamble With Your Health
Be Proactive – Use a Shower Filter

The most effective method of removing these hazards from your shower is the quick and easy installation of a filter on your shower arm. The filter we found to be the best removes chlorine, lead, mercury, iron, chlorine by-products, arsenic, hydrogen sulfide, and many other unseen contaminants, such as bacteria, fungi, dirt and sediments. It has a 12 to 18 month filter life-span and the filter can be easily cleaned by backwashing and replaced when needed. I have been using an approved shower filter for many years and really enjoy my chlorine-free showers! Start enjoying safe, chlorine-free showers right away. It's essential to help reduce your risk of heart disease and cancer and to ease the strain on your immune system. And you may even get rid of any long-standing conditions – from sinus and respiratory problems to dry, itchy skin.

Dr. Mercola's 10-Point Shower Filter Checklist

Here's the selection checklist my team and I used to help us search for the best shower filters. To be considered for regular use, the shower filtration system must:

- Filter out a high majority of chlorine
- Filter out the vast majority of chlorine by-products, in particular trihalomethanes (THMs)
- Remove other VOCs (volatile organic compounds)
- Reduce heavy metals – especially lead and copper
- Employ a multi-stage filtering system
- Provide smooth water flow – filtering system needs to be designed so it does not clog
- Deliver a system that's easy to install
- Look attractive and be practical to maintain
- Be reasonably priced
- Show proof of manufacturer's commitment to quality

Little things are like weeds – the longer we neglect them, the larger they grow.

Ten Common-Sense Reasons Why You Should Only Drink Pure, Distilled Water!

- There are over 12,000 chemicals on the market today . . . and 500 are being added annually! Regardless of where you live – in the city or on the farm, some of these chemicals are getting into your drinking water.

- No one knows what effects these toxic chemicals may have upon the body and what and how many toxic combinations are created. Example: It's like making a mixture of colors; just one drop can change the color.

- No equipment has been designed to detect these harmful chemical combinations and may not be for years.

- The body is made up of approximately 75% water, the essential fluid of life. Therefore, don't you think you should be wise about the type of water you drink?

- The U.S. Navy has been drinking distilled water for years!

- Distilled water is chemical and mineral free. Distillation removes all the chemicals and impurities from water that are possible to remove. If the distillation method doesn't remove them, there is no method known today that will.

- The body does need minerals, but it's not necessary that they come from water. There is not one mineral in water which cannot be found more abundantly in food! Water is the most unreliable source of minerals because it varies from one area to another. The food we eat – not the water we drink – is our best reliable source of organic minerals!

- Distilled water is used for intravenous feeding, inhalation therapy, prescriptions and baby formulas. Therefore, doesn't it make common sense that distilled water is good and healthier for everyone to use as their drinking water?

- Thousands of water distillers have been sold throughout the United States and many foreign countries to individuals, families, dentists, doctors, hospitals, nursing homes and government agencies and these informed, alert consumers are helping protect their health by using only pure distilled water. They don't want toxic chemicals!

- With all the pollutants and minerals, including chemicals and other toxic impurities in our water, it makes good sense to clean it up the safest, most efficient and least expensive way, with the best distillation process.

Distilled Water Questions and Answers

Q. We have recently installed a home water softener. Is this good, pure drinking water?

A. No, don't drink it! (pages 52 and 108-114) Water softeners don't eliminate inorganic minerals, but merely hold them in suspension in an ionized state. It makes more soapsuds – but leaves inorganic mineral deposits in your home and human plumbing to cause problems!

Q. Will distilled water help my complexion?

A. Yes – distilled water helps you have a smooth, firmer, radiant complexion in 2 ways – by drinking it for internal cleanliness and by cleansing your skin with it externally. Hard water seals the pores and tends to clog them. **Use an Apple Cider Vinegar Facial Tonic Spray:** for men and women, spray or pat on face (50% ACV & 50% distilled water mixture, it's refreshing cold – keep in refrigerator) daily for amazing results!

Q. I have an obesity problem. Will drinking distilled water help me to lose weight?

159

A. Yes – drinking 8 glasses of distilled water daily is filling and adding 2 tsps of raw organic apple cider vinegar to 3 of them (recipe page 130) promotes detox cleansing and cuts desire for sweets and heavy foods. Also eliminate salt from your diet! A primary symptom of obesity is retention of fluid. A major cause of waterlogged tissues is due to the fact that table salt, composed of sodium chloride, is an inorganic mineral which is indigestible by the human body and is held in solution with water. Hard water makes this condition worse by adding more indigestible inorganic minerals, further impairing the body's system of elimination. Ample distilled water helps the body function better in every way, including the better elimination of accumulated harmful and inorganic toxins. Distilled water is especially good to detox your liver and kidneys, which are the organs most abused by salt and hard water, inorganic minerals, fluorides, chlorides, etc.

The natural healing force within us is the greatest force in getting well. – Hippocrates, The Father of Medicine

Distilled Water Questions and Answers

Q. Is distilled water recommended for babies?

A. Yes, it's not only recommended, it's prescribed for babies! Distilled water should be used internally for formulas, food, etc., also externally for cleaning babies. Diaper rash and skin problems can result from hard water deposits and chemicals even on sheets, clothes, and diapers. Do the final rinse in distilled water.

Q. Can animals and wildlife tell the difference between hard and distilled water?

A. Yes. Place a variety of waters before a goat, for example, and he will select distilled water. Use it in your bird bath and the birds will return yearly. Many a race has been lost because trainers didn't provide their thoroughbreds with distilled purified water.

Q. Does hard water affect everyone the same way?

A. No. All human systems are basically similar, but no two are exactly alike! Mineral deposits from hard water tend to migrate to the body's weakest points: the intestinal walls, causing constipation; creating gallbladder and kidney stones; in the arteries, leading to arteriosclerosis; in the joints, inviting arthritis; etc.

Of course, when the functions of any one part of the body are impaired, the entire system is affected and gradually weakened! Thus, multiple symptoms appear as evidence of more widespread systematic damage. Your best insurance against all these symptoms of "ageing" is to drink distilled water.

Q. Do athletes drink distilled water?

A. Many famous ones do. Connie Mack, 50 years the Philadelphia Athletics manager, would not allow his players to drink hard water – and he had champion healthy teams. Connie Mack also "practiced what he preached" and maintained his own perfect health past 90. We have heard of lots of champion teams in all sports and Olympic and Triathlete Champions as well who follow the Bragg Healthy Lifestyle and drink pure distilled water!

160

We love helping people who want to live and follow
The Bragg Healthy Lifestyle! We want to help you now!

Wise Water Saving Tips To Use:

Saving water is easy. There are a number of ways to save water, and they all start with you. Here are a few suggestions from *www.WaterUseItWisely.com.*

- Don't leave the water running when doing the dishes.
- Take shallow baths and quick showers (5 minutes saves up to 1,000 gallons a month).
- Install low-flow shower heads and water-saving aerators on all your faucets.
- Use a broom to clean instead of hosing down sidewalks and driveways.
- Water your lawn in early mornings or late evenings.
- Flush fresh water toilets only as needed.
- Fix all leaky water faucets and pipes!
- When doing laundry, match the size of the load to the water level.
- If you drop an ice cube, don't throw it in the sink, drop it in a houseplant instead.
- Use a car wash that recycles water.

Please Conserve Water, visit: WaterUseItWisely.com

What is Your Water Footprint?

Now you can calculate your personal water footprint: a set of brief questions that will get you thinking about how much water you and your household use and how water connects to almost every aspect of your life! The calculator will help you explore how you use water, estimate your household's water footprint and learn ways to conserve. – See web: *gracelinks.org/1408/water-footprint-calculator.*

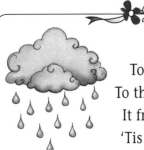

DISTILLED WATER
To the days of the aged it addeth length;
To the might of the strong it addeth strength;
It freshens the heart, it brightens the sight;
'Tis like quaffing a goblet of morning light.

THE MIRACLES OF APPLE CIDER VINEGAR FOR A STRONGER, LONGER, HEALTHIER LIFE

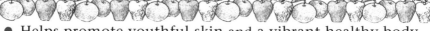

> *The old adage is true:*
> *"An apple a day*
> *keeps the doctor away."*

- Helps promote youthful skin and a vibrant healthy body
- Helps remove artery plaque, infections and body toxins
- Helps fight germs, viruses, bacteria and mold naturally
- Helps retard old age onset in humans, pets and farm animals
- Helps regulate calcium metabolism
- Helps keep blood the right consistency
- Helps regulate women's menstruation, relieves PMS, and UTI
- Helps normalize urine pH, relieving frequent urge to urinate
- Helps digestion, assimilation and helps balance the pH
- Helps protect against food poisoning and even brings relief if you do get it
- Helps relieve sore throats, laryngitis and throat tickles and cleans out throat mucus and gum toxins
- Helps detox the body so sinus, asthma and flu sufferers can breathe easier and more normally
- Helps banish acne, athlete's foot, soothes burns, sunburns
- Helps prevent itching scalp, dandruff, and dry hair
- Helps fight arthritis and helps remove crystals and toxins from joints, tissues, organs and entire body
- Helps control and normalize body weight

162

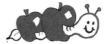

– Paul C. Bragg, N.D., Ph.D., Health Crusader,
Originator of Health Stores

Our sincere blessings to you, dear friends, who make our lives so worthwhile and fulfilled by reading our teachings on natural living as our Creator laid down for us to follow. He wants us to follow the simple path of natural living. This is what we teach in our books and health crusades worldwide. Our prayers reach out to you and your loved ones for the best in health and happiness. We must follow the laws He has laid down for us, so we can reap this precious health physically, mentally, emotionally and spiritually!

HAVE AN APPLE HEALTHY LIFE!   *With Love,*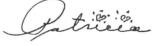

 Raw organic, unfiltered apple cider vinegar with the "Mother Enzyme" is #1 food I recommend to stop heartburn, gerd, gas, indigestion and for maintaining body's vital acid-alkaline balance and digestion. – Gabriel Cousens, M.D., Author, "Conscious Eating"

Chapter 11

ENVIRONMENT & POLLUTION

Since its first publication, *Water – The Shocking Truth* has been in such demand that the last printing was almost sold out the day it was printed! Now it's in the 31st printing, we feel, it is playing an important part in the development of widespread public awareness of Mother Earth's environmental water, soil and air problems. Man is finally realizing that he cannot continue to contaminate this planet Earth and survive! This Special Supplement serves to brings you even more important information on this vital subject of pure water.

A New Era of Personal Ecology

The damage to our natural resources has become personalized in the form of a terrible threat to our health and our very lives. Technology has outstripped biology! The increasing mechanization and industrialization of our society – at first welcomed as benefactors bringing creature comforts and labor-saving devices – are now revealed as "Trojan Horses" bringing the various toxic enemies into our very homes that can destroy us!

163

Biochemists Shocked by Lab Tests

Biochemists are alarmed by the result of laboratory tests which reveal increasing deposits of inorganic "heavy metals" in our human bodies. The dangerous effects of the increasing pollution of our water, soil, food and air are evidenced by the fact that:

- 90% of tests show mercury poisoning.
- 85% of tests show lead intoxication.
- 37% of tests show arsenic poisoning.
- 70% of tests show zinc accumulations.

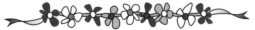

Water from chemically treated public water systems – even from many wells and springs – is likely to be loaded with poisonous chemicals and toxic trace elements.

Destiny is not a matter of chance; it is a matter of choice. It is not a thing to be waited for, it is a thing to be achieved. – William Jennings Bryan

Many Are Poisoned By Food and Water

Mercury . . . lead . . . arsenic . . . zinc . . . none of us deliberately take these inorganic mineral poisons into our systems. Or do we? How could we? Health-minded people drink distilled water, organic fruit and vegetable juices, and try to eat only organically grown foods.

The tragic truth about the water and organic foods and juices is that even these substances can become contaminated, because so much of our air, water and soil are contaminated by industrial and agricultural pollutants. We are aware of radioactive fallout and have demanded safeguards against it. But what about the daily fallout of inorganic wastes from factory exhausts? What about poisonous pesticides, chemical fertilizers and the deadly food additives put into American foods?

Rain water, for example, was once and rightly so considered pure – but no longer! Pure it may be when it leaves the clouds. But if it passes through air polluted by industrial and automotive toxic wastes – including everything from sooty carbons to strontium, arsenic, selenium, beryllium, copper, lead, mercury and fluorides – it should be labeled "hazardous to your health!"

164

When these poisons, especially the deadly fluoride gases, are absorbed by the soil it also becomes toxic. Add to this the toxic contaminants contained in poisonous pesticides and chemical fertilizers that large industrial farms and growers use to increase crop production. Grains, vegetables and fruits will absorb these poisons and so will meat from animals that feed on contaminated grass and feed. It's no wonder millions of people are only half-alive, suffering with physical health problems!

Please Take Action Today! Everyone is at Risk!

Rachel Carson's call for active involvement in our environment is still an absolute necessity! As the tide of chemicals born in the Industrial Age has arisen to engulf our environment, a drastic change has come about in the nature of the most serious public health problem. For the first time in the history of the world, every human being is now subject to many dangerous chemicals, from the moment of conception until death. – Rachel Carson, author – "Silent Spring", 1962

GMO Soybeans & Glyphosate Cancer Link

An alarming study in "Food and Chemical Toxicology" journal finds that *glyphosate*, the world's most widely used herbicide and weed-killer is capable of driving estrogen receptor breast cancer cells to multiply. The researchers also discovered that the naturally occurring *phytoestrogen* in soybeans (known as *genistein*) produced "an additive estrogenic effect" when combined with glyphosate, raising the question as to whether GMO soybeans are contributing to the epidemic levels of breast cancer within the U.S. where they are consumed in relatively high quantities. *This study implied that the additive effect of glyphosate and genistein in women may induce cancer cell growth.*

Glyphosate Pollution is Now Everywhere!

One study found glyphosate in 60-100% of all U.S. air and rain samples tested and another study found that glyphosate widely contaminates groundwater. Glyphosate is acutely toxic to fish, frogs and birds and can kill beneficial insects and soil organisms that maintain ecological balance. Numerous studies have also shown that glyphosate is contributing to the huge increase in plant and crop diseases! It is therefore impossible to seal yourself off from the growing global environmental threats.

Help Reduce Water Pollution and Runoff

Every household activity contributes to our water pollution. When it rains, fertilizer from lawns, oil from driveways, paint and solvent residues from walls and decks and even pet waste are all washed into storm sewers, nearby lakes, rivers, and streams – *the same lakes, rivers and streams we rely on for our drinking water supply!*

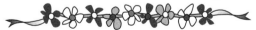

Glyphosate is a herbicide used in agriculture and aquatic systems. Exposure to it may occur from its normal use due to drift, residues in food crops and from runoff into potential drinking water sources.

Trees help to reduce storm water runoff. They can beautify landscapes and absorb excess carbon dioxide. Water is also taken up by roots so less runs off goes into the lakes, streams and ocean.

Here are ten ways to help reduce water pollution run-off:

1. Decrease hard surfaces such as concrete and asphalt and landscape with vegetation to decrease run-off.
2. Use native plants and natural fertilizer such as compost and peat to help retain soil moisture.
3. Don't over-water lawns and gardens.
4. Recycle and dispose of trash properly.
5. Correctly dispose of hazardous household products such as paint, used oil, cleaning solvents, chemicals, etc.
6. Use non-toxic household products whenever possible.
7. Recycle used motor oil.
8. Be "green" when washing car. Go to a car wash. They are required to drain their wastewater into sewer system. Also many car washes recycle their wastewater, and use less than half the amount used at home.
9. Help identify, report and stop polluters.
10. Be an activist. Educate yourself. Contact your public officials. Go to hearings, support laws to protect our water. Volunteer for coastal clean-up or tree planting.

166

Political Action for Permanent Ecology

Politicians, in response to heightened public opinions, have made many promises to help clean up the environment. Some issues: GMOs, urban air pollution, and chemtrails are discussed, but sadly the U.S. and planetary ecology is still dangerously corrupted (air and water radiation see *RadiationNetwork.com)* not to mention climate change and global warming.

It seems that each time we meet one challenge another comes along! New chemicals are introduced almost daily that threaten our health! These attack our food and water. Our drinking water sources – rivers, lakes and oceans, are becoming contaminated far beyond established safe, healthy levels! We must take action to ensure good health for ourselves and families even as worldwide scientific institutions sadly agree we are in danger of continuing to poison the earth and ourselves. Some have offered sober warnings, even countdown time tables! So far these warnings have only generated token action by governments. Please protest to your congressman or representative, see web: *usa.gov/elected-officials*

But there is one voice that every politician heeds – the combined voice of aroused voters who demand action! This is the one sound that rises above the clink of campaign contributions from big money industrial, agricultural, manufacturing, financial and business interests. To achieve the desired effect – political action on any and all levels – the voice of the voters must be strong, widespread, more aroused and united in purpose.

What Can One Person Do? – Miracles!

Whether you are counting to 10 or to a million, you have to begin with one! That's how political action starts. Begin with yourself, your family, friends and neighbors, involve your clubs, church and other groups, and write letters to editors of local newspapers. Call, email or write local radio and TV stations. Go to town council meetings and state your health concerns! Visit: *www.senate.gov.*

After you get your hometown or community involved, extend your action into the county, state, and nation! Write, visit, email and call county officials, state officials and your congressmen and women, and even the President and Vice-President of the United States! Don't settle for promises! Demand action – and persist until you get it! It is up to each and every one of us to bring all possible political pressure to bear upon our political leaders to clean up our environment (*water, air, soil*) and restore the world's vital natural ecology. This is what we all must faithfully do – it is our responsibility if we hope to survive this 21st Century!!

167

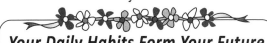

Your Daily Habits Form Your Future

Habits can be wrong, good or bad, healthy or unhealthy, rewarding or unrewarding. The right or wrong habits, decisions, actions, words or deeds . . . are up to you! Wisely choose your habits, as they can make or break your life! – Patricia Bragg

The body and mind are so closely connected that not even a single word or thought can come into existence without being reflected in the personality & health of the individual. – John Holmes Prentiss, 1784-1861

We all grow healthier in nature, gentle sunshine and love! – Patricia Bragg

Test Your Water – Drink Safe Water

With so many of American water supplies contaminated by harmful chemicals and toxic additives, how can we make sure that we provide only safe, healthful water for ourselves and our families? One relatively simple answer is to drink only distilled bottled water. But even this method requires care, for not all bottled water lives up to even FDA bottled water standards. Before you buy any bottled water ask for an analysis – it's your right and it's your health at risk! Let's work to prevent these water atrocities and get quick action to clean up our country's precious water supplies!!! Call or write to your bottled water company and city water board to demand proof that your water supply contains no THMs (trihalomethanes, also formed through chlorination), carcinogens, fluoride and other synthetic or organic chemicals and pesticides! Get your water tested! Call your Public Health Department for details. This website will help you test your home water, well, stream, etc. Visit web: *e-watertest.com*

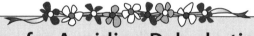

Tips for Avoiding Dehydration:

Dehydration happens when your body loses or uses more fluids than it takes in. When this happens, your body isn't able to do all the things it's supposed to. It's especially dangerous in older people and young children.

1. **Pay attention to the possible signs of dehydration:** headaches, fatigue, vomiting, and you may also feel more irritable and like your energy has been zapped.

2. **Respond to thirst when the feeling strikes.**

3. **Check your urine color.** Your urine color should be clear or a straw color, as opposed to a darker yellow or brown. A dark yellow color is a definite sign of dehydration. Drink water right away!

4. **Eat hydrating foods throughout the day.** Melons and berries have a particularly high water content, helping you stay hydrated. (Remember, sugary drinks can lead to weight gain and inflammation, which can increase your risk for diabetes.)

www.everydayhealth.com/dehydration/prevention

Protector of Our Oceans, Sea Life and Waters
Wyland, Famous Whale Wall Artist

As a young man from Michigan, Wyland saw a pair of whales barely 100 yards offshore on his first Pacific Ocean visit. He was so inspired that he has devoted the rest of his life to creating art that captures the beauty of these magnificent creatures. It has been more than 40 years since Wyland began painting his landmark marine life murals. Wyland has a passion for whales and the oceans and is inspired to make a difference in the world. He has painted 100 Walls which equals 16,302 feet of murals (3.1 miles). He completed Whaling Wall #100 in July 2008 for the Olympics in China, where he painted nearly one mile of canvas with kids from Olympic and U.N. member countries. He created a 4,000-square foot painting entitled, "Earth: The Blue Planet," for the world premier of Disney-

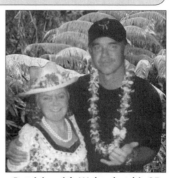

Patricia with Wyland at his 25 year celebration of creating Whale Walls. Wyland follows The Bragg Healthy Lifestyle and has super energy and health.

Nature's first feature film, *EARTH*. He painted the largest painting of Earth on top of the Long Beach Sports Arena in celebration of Earth Day 2009. He launched FOCUS (Forests, Ocean, Climate – and Us) in partnership with the US Forest

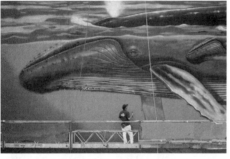

169

Service and National Oceanographic and Atmospheric Administration (NOAA) to educate children about the interconnectedness of our natural resources (water) and habitats.

Patricia shares in Wylands commitment to the protection and preservation of the world's waters and the abundant life within them. To learn more about Wyland and his great artwork, visit his website: *www.wyland.com*

100 Wyland Whale Walls Worldwide

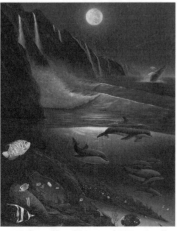

Wyland's "Sacred Waters"

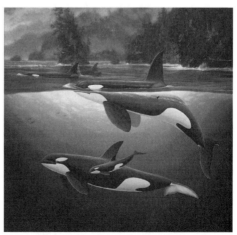

Wyland's "Northern Waters"

HEALTHY HEART HABITS FOR LONG, VITAL LIFE

Remember, *organic live foods make live people. You are what you eat, drink, breathe, think, say and do.* So eat a low-fat, low-sugar, high-fiber diet of organic fresh raw salads, sprouts, greens, vegetables, whole grains, fruits, raw seeds, nuts, fresh juices and chemical-free, purified or distilled water.

Earn your food with daily exercise. For regular exercise, brisk walking, improves your health, stamina, go-power, flexibility, endurance and helps open the cardiovascular system! Only 45 minutes a day truly can do miracles for your heart, arteries, mind, nerves, soul and body! You become revitalized with new zest for living to accomplish your life goals!

We are made of tubes. To help keep them open, clean and to maintain good elimination, I take 1 veg psyllium cap or add 1 tsp psyllium husk powder daily an hour after dinner to juices, herbal teas, even apple cider vinegar drink. I also take one Cayenne capsule (40,000 HU) daily with a meal. I also take 50 to 100 mgs. regular-released Niacin (B3) with one meal daily to help cleanse and open the cardiovascular system; also improves memory. Skin flushing may occur, don't worry about this as it shows it's working! After cholesterol level reaches 180, then only take Niacin twice weekly.

The heart needs healthy balanced nutrients, so take natural multi-vitamin-mineral food supplements: Omega-3 and extra heart helpers – vitamin E with mixed tocotrienols; vitamin C; Ubiquinol CoQ10; vitamin D3; MSM; D-Ribose; garlic; turmeric; selenium; zinc; beta carotene and amino acids – L-Carnitine, L-Taurine, L-Lysine and Proline. Folic acid, CoQ10, vitamin B6 and B12 helps keep homocysteine level low. Magnesium orotate, hawthorn berry extract helps bring relief for palpitations, arrhythmia, senile hearts and coronary disease. Take multi-digestive enzyme and probiotics with meals; it aids in digestion, assimilation and elimination.

For sleep problems try 5-HTP tryptophan (an amino acid), melatonin, calcium, magnesium, valerian (in capsule, extract or tea), and Sleepytime herb tea. For arthritis or joint pain/stiffness, try aloe juice or gel, glucosamine-chondroitin-MSM combo caps and shots, helps heal and regenerate. Capsaicin and DMSO lotion helps relieve pain. Natural liver cleanses to repair and regenerate include: milk thistle; dandelion root; artichoke and turmeric. Dandelion root is a natural diuretic and helps clear toxins through urination and also helps stimulate liver bile flow so waste can be eliminated.

Use amazing antioxidants – E Tocotrienols, vitamin C, quercetin, grape seed extract (OPCs), CoQ10, selenium, SOD, resveratrol, and alpha-lipoic acid. They improve immune system and help flush out dangerous free radicals that cause havoc with cardiovascular pipes and health. Research shows antioxidants promote longevity, slow ageing, fight toxins, help prevent disease, cancer, cataracts and exhaustion.

Recommended Heart Health Tests (for Adults):

- **Total Cholesterol:** 180 mg/dl or less is optimal
- **LDL Cholesterol:** 130 mg/dl or less is optimal • **HDL Cholesterol:** 50 mg/dl or more
- **Triglycerides:** 150 mg/dl or less is normal level
- **HDL/Cholesterol Ratio:** 5.0 or less • **Triglycerides/HDL Ratio:** below 2
- **Homocysteine:** 6-9 micromoles/L
- **CRP (C-Reactive Protein high sensitivity):**
    - 1 mg/L = low risk • 1-3 mg/L = average risk • over 3 mg/L = high risk
- **Diabetic Risk Tests:**
    - **Glucose:** (do 12 hour food fast) 80-100 mg/dl • **Hemoglobin A1c:** 6% or less
- **Blood Pressure:** 120/70 mmHg is good for adults

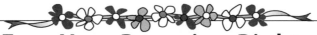

Earn Your Bragging Rights
Live The Bragg Healthy Lifestyle
To Attain Supreme Physical, Mental,
Emotional and Spiritual Health!

With your new awareness, understanding and sincere commitment of how to live The Bragg Healthy Lifestyle!

God bless you and your family and may He give you the strength, the courage and the patience to win your battle to re-enter the Healthy Garden of Eden while you are still living here on Earth with more years to enjoy it all!

With Blessings of Health, Peace, Joy and Love,

Paul and *Patricia*

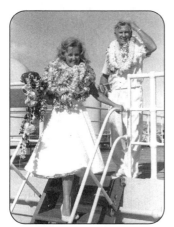

Health Crusaders Paul C. Bragg and daughter Patricia traveled the world spreading health, inspiring millions to renew and revitalize their health.

171

The Bragg books are written to inspire and guide you to health, fitness and longevity. Remember, the book you don't read won't help. So please reread Bragg Books and live The Bragg Healthy Lifestyle to enjoy a healthy fulfilled life!

I never suspected that I would have to learn how to live – that there were specific disciplines and ways of seeing the world that I had to master before I could awaken to a simple, healthy, happy, uncomplicated life. – Dan Millman, author "The Way of the Peaceful Warrior" • peacefulwarrior.com A Bragg fan and admirer since his Stanford University coaching days.

A truly good book teaches me better than to just read it, I must soon lay it down and commence living in its wisdom. What I began by reading, I must finish by acting! – Henry David Thoreau

FROM THE AUTHORS

This book was written for You! It can be your passport to a healthy, long, vital life. We in the Alternative Health Therapies join hands in one common objective – promoting a high standard of health for everyone. Healthy nutrition points the way – which is Mother Nature and God's Way. This book teaches you how to work with them, not against them! Health doctors, therapists nurses, teachers and caregivers are becoming more dedicated than ever before to keeping their patients healthy and fit. This book was written to emphasize the greatly needed importance of healthy lifestyle living for health and longevity, close to Mother Nature and God.

Statements in this book are scientific health findings, known facts of physiology and biological therapeutics. Paul C. Bragg practiced natural methods of living for over 80 years with highly beneficial results, knowing they were safe and of great value. His daughter Patricia lectured and co-authored Bragg Health Books with him and continues carrying on The Bragg Healthy Lifestyle.

Paul C. Bragg and daughter Patricia express their opinions solely as Public Health Educators and Health Crusaders. They offer no cure for disease. Only the body has the ability to cure a person. Experts may disagree with some of the statements made in this book. However, such statements are considered to be factual, based on the long-time experience of dedicated pioneer Health Crusaders Paul C. Bragg and Patricia Bragg. If you suspect you have a medical problem, please always seek qualified Health Care professionals to help you make the healthiest, wisest and best-informed choices!

Count your blessings daily while you do your 30 to 45 minute brisk walks and exercises with these affirmations – health! strength! youth! vitality! peace! laughter! humility! understanding! forgiveness! joy! and love for eternity! and soon all these qualities will come flooding and bouncing into your life. With blessings of super health, peace and love to you, our dear friends – our readers. – Patricia Bragg, Health Crusader

If I were to name the three most precious resources of life, I would say books, friends and nature; and the greatest of these, at least the most constant and always at hand is Mother Nature and God. – John Burroughs

Books to Read on Dangers of Fluoride

Fluoridation: Errors and Omissions in Experimental Trials, Sutton, Phillip, R.N. Melbourne University Press, 1960.

Fluoride: Drinking Ourselves to Death?, Groves, Barry, A. Newleaf, 2002. (great research)

Fluoride the Aging Factor: How to Recognize and Avoid the Devastating Effects of Fluoride, Yiamouyiannis, John, M.D. Health Action Press, 3rd edition, June 1993.

The Case Against Fluoride: How Hazardous Waste Ended Up in Our Drinking Water and the Bad Science and Powerful Politics That Keep It There, Connett, Paul, Ph.D., Beck, James, M.D., Ph.D., Micklem, H.S., D.Phil, Chelsea Green Publishing, 1st edition, October 2010.

The Devil's Poison: How Fluoride is Killing You, Murphy, Dean. Trafford Publishing, 2008.

173

The Fluoride Deception, Bryson, Christopher. Seven Stories Press, 2004. (great exposé and research on fluoride)

The Fluoride Question: Panacea or Poison?, Gotzsche, Anne-Lise. Stein and Day, 1st edition, 1975.

The Greatest Fraud: Fluoridation, Sutton, Philip, R.N. Kurunda Pty. Ltd., 1994. Available: *www.whale.to/d/sutton_b.html*

Articles & Editorials on Toxic Fluoride

Burgstahler, A.W. and Colquhoun, J., "Neurotoxicity of fluoride." *Fluoride*, Vol. 29:57-8, 1996.

Cohn, P.D., "A brief report on the association of drinking water fluoridation and the incidence of osteosarcoma among young males." New Jersey Department of Health, November 8, 1992. See web: *www.slweb.org/cohn-1992.html*

Colquhoun, J., "Disfiguring dental fluorosis in Auckland, New Zealand." *Fluoride*, Vol. 17:66-72, 1984.

Cooper, C., Wickham, C.A.C., Barker, D.J.R. and Jacobsen, S.J., "Water fluoridation and hip fracture" (letter). *Journal of the American Medical Association*, Vol. 266:513, 1991.

Articles & Editorials on Toxic Fluoride

Czerwinski, E., et al, "Bone and joint pathology in fluoride-exposed workers." *Archives of Environmental Health*, Vol. 43:340-3, September/October 1988.

Danielson, C., Lyon, J.L., Egger, M. and Goodenough, G.K., "Hip fractures and fluoridation in Utah's elderly population."*Journal of the American Medical Association,* Vol. 286:746-8, 1992.

Foulkes, R.G., "Celebration or Shame? 50 Years of Fluoridation (1945-1995)." *Townsend Letter for Doctors and Patients,* Nov. 1995. See web: *sonic.net/kryptox/medicine/foulkes2.htm*

Freni, S.C., "Exposure to high fluoride concentration in drinking water is associated with decreased birth rates." *Journal of Toxicology & Environmental Health,* Vol. 42:109-121, 1994. See web: *FluorideAlert.org/studies/fertility01*

Gessner, B.D., "Acute fluoride poisoning from a public water system." *New England Journal of Medicine,* Vol. 330:95-99, 1994.

Hedlund, L.R. and Gallagher, J.C., "Increased incidence of hip fracture in osteoporotic women treated with sodium fluoride." *Journal of Bone and Mineral Research,* Vol. 4:223-5, 1989.

Hileman, B., "Fluoridation of water. Questions about health risks and benefits remain after more than forty years." *Chemical and Engineering News,* Vol. 66:26-42, August 1988.

Jacobsen, S.J., et al, "Regional variation in the incidence of hip fracture." *Journal of the American Medical Association,* Vol. 264:500-502, 1990.

Jacobsen, S.J., O'Fallon, W.M., Melton, L.J., 3rd, "Hip fracture incidence before and after the fluoridation of the public water supply, Rochester, Minnesota." *American Journal of Public Health,* Vol. 83:743-5, May 1993.

Leverett, D.H., "Prevalence of dental fluorosis in fluoridated and non-fluoridated communities – preliminary investigation." *Journal of Public Health Dentistry,* Vol. 46:184-7, 1986.

Mahoney, M.C., et al, "Bone cancer incidence rates in New York State: time trends and fluoridated water." *American Journal of Public Health,* Vol. 81:475-9, April 1991.

Masuda, T.T., "Persistence of fluoride from organic origins in waste waters." *Developments in Industrial Microbiology,* Vol. 5:53-70, 1964. See web: *FluorideAlert.org/articles/groth-1975*

Sowers, M.R., et al, "The relationship of bone mass and fracture history to fluoride and calcium intake: a study of three communities." *American Journal of Clinical Nutrition,* Vol. 44:889-98, 1986. Web: *ajcn.nutrition.org/content/44/6.toc*

Sowers, M.R., Clerk, K.M., Jannausch, M.L., and Wallace, R.B., "A prospective study of bone mineral content and fracture in communities with differential fluoride exposure." *American Journal of Epidemiology,* Vol. 133:649-60, April 1991.

Susheela, A.K., et al, "Fluoride ingestion and its correlation with gastrointestinal discomfort." *Fluoride,* Vol. 25: 5-22, 1992.

Waldbott, G.L., Lee, J.R., "Toxicity from repeated low-grade exposure to hydrogen fluoride – case report." *Clinical Toxicology,* Vol. 13:391-402, 1978. See: *slweb.org/chemicals.html*

Yiamouyiannis, J., "Water fluoridation and tooth decay: results from the 1986-1987, National Survey of U.S. school children." *Fluoride,* Vol. 23:55-67, 1990.

Yiamouyiannis, J., "Fluoridation and cancer: the biology and epidemiology of bone and oral cancer related to fluoridation." *Fluoride,* Vol. 26:83-96, 1993.

Zhao, L.B., et al, "Effect of a high fluoride water supply on children's intelligence." *Fluoride,* Vol. 29:190-2, 1996.

U.S. Dept. of Health & Human Services

Agency for Toxic Substances and Disease Registry, "Toxicological Profile for Fluorides, Hydrogen Fluoride, & Fluorine." April 1993.

Contact: Agency for Toxic Substances and Disease Registry

atsdr.cdc.gov/substances/index.asp • 800-232-4636

Websites Recommended on Water Research

Toxic Fluoride and Other Chemicals:

- www.FluorideAlert.org/
- www.LoveTheTruth.com/truth_about_fluoride.htm
- NaturalNews.com/038217_fluoride_tap_water_side_effects.html
- www.nccn.net/~wwithin/fluoride.htm
- www.pure-earth.com/chlorine.html
- www.slweb.org/fluoridation.html
- www.wnho.net/fluoride_news.htm

Water Treatment and Distilled Water:

- www.AquariusTheWaterBearer.com
- GlobalHealingCenter.com/natural-health/3-health-benefits-distilled-water
- lenntech.com/applications/drinking/drinking-water.htm
- www.WaterWise.com

Government Standards for Water:

- water.epa.gov/lawsregs/rulesregs
- doh.wa.gov/Portals/1/Documents/Pubs/331-181.pdf

Water for Health Reasons:

- www.WaterCure.com

Testing and Conserving Water:

- gracelinks.org/1408/water-footprint-calculator
- e-watertest.com
- WaterUseItWisely.com

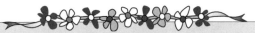

Praises for: *Water – The Shocking Truth*

"In my opinion, *Water – The Shocking Truth* is destined to become a landmark – not just in the field of so-called health literature – but particularly in the field of standard internal medicine. Following a massive coronary thrombosis 13 years ago, I have been on a strict regimen of distilled water, health diet, vitamin therapy and exercise – and the results have exceeded my expectations. I feel better at 67 than I did at 47. My arteries are clean and healthy; my joints have limbered; my vision is sharper; my nerves are calmer; and my head is clearer. My own experience corroborates your findings. I am convinced that distilled water has been the most important facet of my rejuvenation program."

– Ben H. Martin, California

I developed painful arthritis in my hands and had to stop playing my violin. I read your water book and started drinking 8 glasses of distilled water daily adding a tablespoon of your organic apple cider vinegar to 3 of them. I am totally cured.

– Geraldine Boundey, California

"One of the greatest things that ever happened to me was attending your health classes 35 years ago in Miami, Florida. Thanks to your teachings, I am now 57 years young and love living The Bragg Healthy Lifestyle!! I have read all of the Bragg books many times, and have just finished the sixth reading of your *Water* book. To me this is the greatest book! Keep up the crusading!"

– Cliff Hayes, Florida

It's the song you sing and the smiles you wear,
that's making the sunshine everywhere.
– James Whitcomb Riley

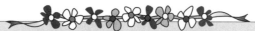

Praises for: *Water – The Shocking Truth*

"Thank you for your fine review of my books, *Hunza Land* and *The Choice Is Clear.* And let me repeat my thanks to you for your great book, *Water – The Shocking Truth,* which I recommend as a 'must' to all my patients. In connection with this subject, I would like to emphasize that a vital factor in the amazing longevity of the people (many over 110–120) of Hunza Land is distilled water. They eat most of their fruits and vegetables raw, raised in organic soil. Fruits and vegetables, of course, are 90% distilled water – nature's own distillation, as you say. Along with that, they drink glacier water, which is low in inorganic minerals. Their main beverage is an organic grape drink, which again is distilled water. So the intake, in isolated Hunza Land of distilled water is 90% greater than that of our modern western civilization."

– Dr. Allen E. Banik, Nebraska, author of:
Hunza Land and *Choice is Clear*

178

"As outlined in your book, *Water – The Shocking Truth,* I know that the closer to nature we can get, the better off we are going to be . . . I am a farmer in Missouri, and have not used any chemicals of any kind on this farm for 15 years, as I came to realize that we should not try to improve on nature, but work with her! I am so happy to find people like you and Patricia, who are not trying to keep the truth to yourselves. You are true health crusaders leading people toward healthy long lives."

– Eugene Kling, Missouri

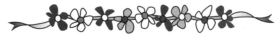

We are recharged and blessed by each one of you reading our health books filled with loving health guidance for our readers – thank you! – Patricia Bragg

---

A book is a garden, an orchard, a storehouse, a party, a mentor, a teacher, a guidepost, and a counsellor. – Henry Ward Beecher

BRAGG PHOTO GALLERY

PATRICIA & PAUL C. BRAGG, N.D., Ph.D.
Dynamic Daughter & Father are World Health Crusaders

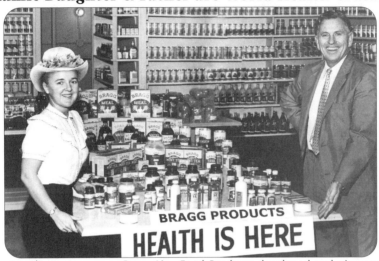

BRAGG PRODUCTS
HEALTH IS HERE

During the past century, Bragg Live Food Products developed and pioneered the very first line of Health Foods, from vitamins and minerals to organic nuts, seeds, and sun-dried fruits. This included over 365 health products, – *"one for each day of the year!"* says daughter Patricia Bragg.

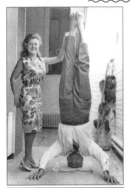

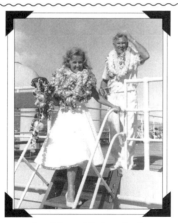

"Thanks for The Bragg Healthy Lifestyle that you shared with me and you are sharing with millions of others worldwide."
– John Gray, Ph.D., author

Picture from
People Magazine August, 1975.

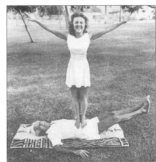

Patricia and father, Paul
on world trip in 1950's,
during stop in Tahiti.

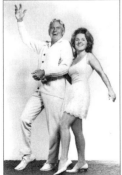

"You have recharged me with joy, hope, love and encouragement, which poured from your words. I am now fasting and using ACV. You have certainly improved my life!"
– Marie Furia, New Jersey

Patricia Bragg stands on her father's stomach. Paul's stomach muscles are so strong he can lift Patricia up and down! **179**

PAUL C. BRAGG, N.D., Ph.D.
HEALTH CRUSADER

Life Extension Specialist and Originator of Health Food Stores

I have experienced a beautiful, remarkable, spiritual and physical awakening since reading Bragg Health Books. I'll never be the same again.
– Sandy Tuttle, Ohio

With every new day comes new strength and new thoughts.
– Eleanor Roosevelt

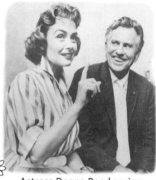

Actress Donna Reed saying "Health First" with Paul C. Bragg.

Dr. Paul C. Bragg (right) Creator Health Food Stores, Pioneer Life Extension Specialist, with his prize student Jack LaLanne. Paul started him on the royal road to health over 85 years ago!

Paul C. Bragg spent much of his time at the Hollywood Studios meeting with top Stars and motion picture industry executives, giving health lectures and private consultations. Dr. Paul C. Bragg was Hollywood's first highly respected, health, fitness and nutrition advisor to the Stars.

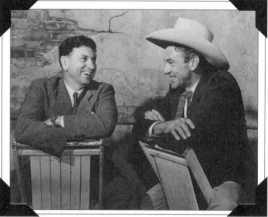

Paul C. Bragg with Gary Cooper, famous American film actor, best known for his many Western films.

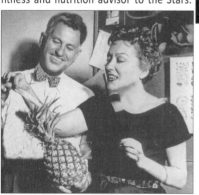

Paul C. Bragg with the famous Hollywood Actress Gloria Swanson, who was leading star in 20s, 30s and 40s. Gloria became a Bragg Health Devotee at 18 and she often would Health Crusade with Bragg during the 1950s.

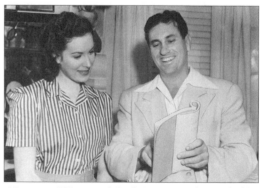

Maureen O'Hara and Paul C. Bragg. This Irish film actress and singer was best noted for playing in "Miracle on 34th Street" and "The Quiet Man."

I'd like to thank you for teaching me how to take control of my health! I lost 55 pounds and I feel "great!" Bragg books have showed me vitality, happiness and being close to Mother Nature. You both are real "Crusaders for Health for the World." Thanks!
– Leonard Amato

Dr. Paul C. Bragg and daughter Patricia were my early guiding inspiration to my health career.
– Jeffery Bland, Ph.D., Famous Food Scientist

The best thing about the future is that it only comes one day at a time.
– Abraham Lincoln

Paul C. Bragg in Tahiti 1920's gathering tropical papaya fruit.

Paul C. Bragg owes his powerful body and superb health to living exclusively on live, vital, healthy, organic rich foods.

Dear Friends – you cannot know how greatly you have impacted my life and some of my friends! We love your Bragg Health Books, teachings and products and are now living healthier, happier lives. Thanks!
– Winnie Brown, Arizona

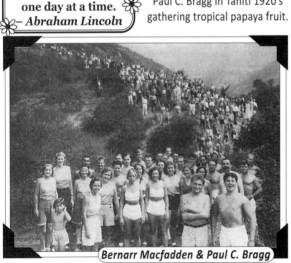

Bernarr Macfadden & Paul C. Bragg

A thousand happy Bragg Health Students enjoy hiking, exercise and fresh air on the trail to Mount Hollywood (above Griffith Observatory) in beautiful California, summer of 1932.

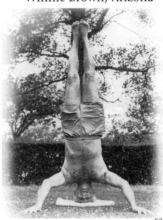

Paul C. Bragg exercising Regent's Park, London.

PAUL & PATRICIA BRAGG

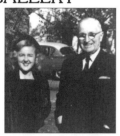

Patricia with 33rd President Harry S. Truman at his home in Independence, Missouri.

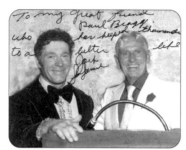

Paul C. Bragg, Creator of Health Food Stores, with his prize student Jack LaLanne, who thanks Bragg for saving his life at 15.

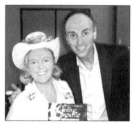

Patrica Bragg with Dr. Jeffrey Smith. He is leader in getting GMO's out of US foods. See GMO video by Jeffrey Smith and narrated by Lisa Oz (Dr. Oz's wife) on web: GeneticRouletteMovie.com

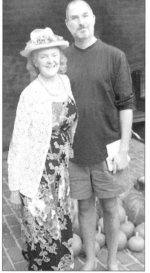

Patricia visiting with Steve Jobs at his home in Palo Alto during the Thanksgiving Holidays.

"I've been reading Bragg Books since high school. I'm thankful for the Bragg Healthy Lifestyle and admire their Health Crusading for a healthier, happier world."
– Steve Jobs, Creator –
Apple Computer

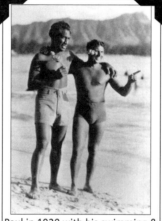

Paul in 1920 with his swimming & surfing friend, Duke Kahanamoku, Waikiki Beach, Diamond Head.

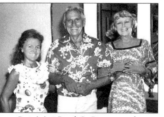

Patricia, Paul C. Bragg and Mrs. Duke (Nadine) Kahanamoku. (Nadine is Patricia's Godmother).

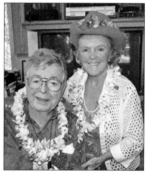

Dr. Earl Bakken with Patricia. He's famous for inventing the first Transistor Pacemaker. His firm Medtronic, developed it and a Resuscitator for fixing ailing hearts that have and are saving thousands of lives. Dr. Bakken lived in Hawaii.

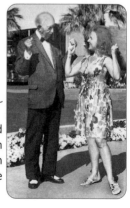

"I cannot remember a time when the Golden Rule was not my motto and precept, the torch that guided my footsteps."* – J.C. Penney

*The Golden Rule: Do unto others as you would have them do unto you.

J.C.Penney & Patricia → exercising. They walked often in Palm Springs when he and his wife visited in the winter to enjoy the warm desert sunshine.

HEALTH CRUSADING TO HOLLYWOOD STARS

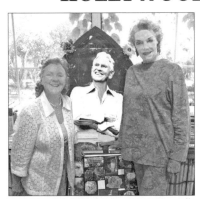

Patricia with friend Actress Jane Russell. Famous Hollywood Star of 40s to 60s.

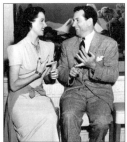

Jane Wyatt learning about health with Paul C. Bragg.

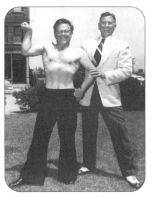

Mickey Rooney with Paul. Rooney was an American film actor and entertainer. He won multiple awards and had one of the longest careers of any actor to age 93!

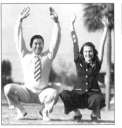

Paul C. Bragg exercising with Actress Helen Parrish.

"Thank you Paul & Patricia Bragg for my simple, easy-to-follow Healthy Lifestyle. You make my days healthy!" – Clint Eastwood, Academy Award Winning Film Producer, Director, Actor and Bragg follower for over 65 years.

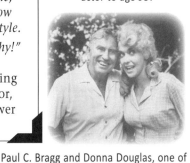

Paul C. Bragg and Donna Douglas, one of Hollywood's most beautiful and talented health advocates. She played the part of "Elly-May" in the Beverly Hillbillies, which became one of the longest-running series in television history and was the #1 show in America in its first 2 years.

Life is a Miracle Minute by Minute Year by Year!

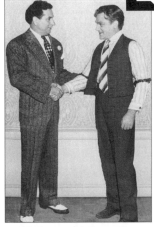

Paul C. Bragg with James Cagney, American film actor. He won major awards for wide variety of roles. The American Film Institute ranked Cagney 8th among the Greatest Male Hollywood Stars of All Time.

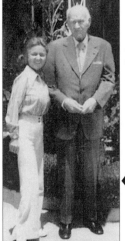

Patricia with Conrad Hilton

← Hotel founder, Conrad Hilton with Patricia Bragg, his Healthy Lifestyle Teacher. *"I wouldn't be alive today if it wasn't for the Braggs and their Bragg Healthy Lifestyle!"* – Conrad Hilton

"Thank you for your website. What a wealth of info to learn about how to live and eat healthy. Many Blessings!" – Michel & Mary, California

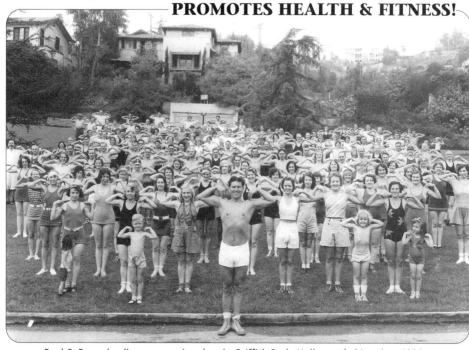

Paul C. Bragg leading an exercise class in Griffith Park, Hollywood, CA – circa 1920s.

Bragg Healthy Lifestyle works Miracles! – Jack LaLanne

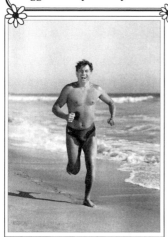

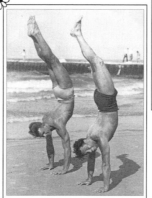

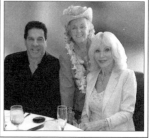

Patricia with Lou and wife Carla at Elaine LaLanne's 90th Birthday Party.

Friend and Paul C. Bragg doing handstand at the beach.

Paul running on Coney Island, New York, where he was a member of the Coney Island Polar Bear Club, known for Cold Water Swimming, 1930s.

TV Hulk Actor Lou Ferrigno gives thanks to Bragg Books. Lou went from puny to become Super Hulk! ➡

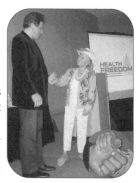

"I lost 102 lbs. with The Bragg Healthy Lifestyle and I have kept it off for over 15 years, staying away from white flour, sugar and other processed foods."
– Dee McCaffrey, Chemist & Diet Counselor, Tempe, AZ

Lou & Patricia in Chicago Health Freedom Expo.

PATRICIA CONTINUING BRAGG HEALTH CRUSADE!

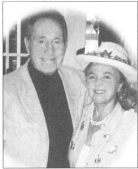

Jack LaLanne with Patricia.

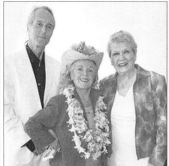

Jon & Elaine LaLanne with Patricia.

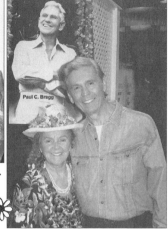

Mother Nature Loves US!

Patricia Bragg with Bill Galt inspired by Bragg Books, he founded Good Earth Restaurants.

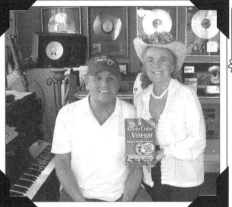

Patricia in studio with famous Beach Boy Bruce Johnston, Bragg follower over 40 years. He played for her their latest records.

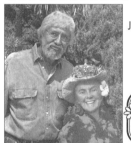

Patricia with Jean-Michel Cousteau Ocean Explorer & Environmentalist. OceanFutures.org

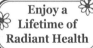

Enjoy a Lifetime of Radiant Health

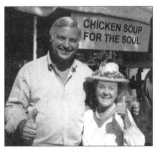

Patricia with Jack Canfield, Bragg follower, Motivational Speaker and Co-Producer of Chicken Soup For The Soul.

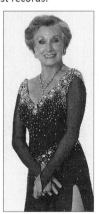

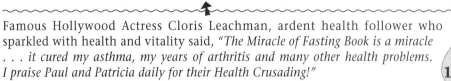

Patricia with Astronaut Buzz Aldrin, celebrating over 50 years since pilot of Apollo 11 first landed on the moon.

Famous Hollywood Actress Cloris Leachman, ardent health follower who sparkled with health and vitality said, *"The Miracle of Fasting Book is a miracle . . . it cured my asthma, my years of arthritis and many other health problems. I praise Paul and Patricia daily for their Health Crusading!"*

PAUL & PATRICIA BRAGG
HEALTH CRUSADING

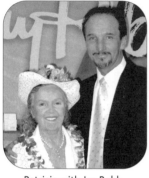

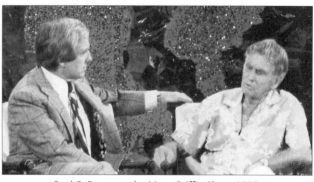

Patricia with Jay Robb.

Paul C. Bragg on the Merv Griffin Show, 1976.

Paul Bragg inspired me many years ago with The Miracle of Fasting Book and his pioneering philosophy on health. His daughter Patricia is a testament to the ageless value of living The Bragg Healthy Lifestyle. – Jay Robb, author of The Fruit Flush

During the many years Patricia worked with her father, she was right beside him, assisting him on Bragg Health Crusades worldwide. They were a great team, when you looked at them, you would see only two people headed in the same healthy direction!

I am a big fan of Paul Bragg. I fast and follow The Bragg Healthy Lifestyle daily. The world and I are blessed with the health teachings of Paul and Patricia Bragg! – Tony Robbins • TonyRobbins.com

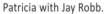

❀ **Dream big,** ❀
think big and enjoy
the many miracles. ❀

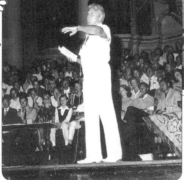

Paul – London Bragg Health Crusade.

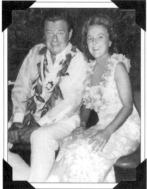

Actor Arthur Godfrey with Patricia, in Honolulu celebrating his 79th birthday.

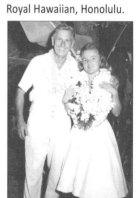

Paul & Daughter Patricia, Royal Hawaiian, Honolulu.

Health Crusaders Paul C. Bragg and daughter Patricia traveled the world spreading health, inspiring millions to renew and revitalize their health.
Bragg Mottos:
3 John 2 and Genesis 6:3

100 YEAR HISTORY OF BRAGG HEALTH BOOKS & PRODUCTS

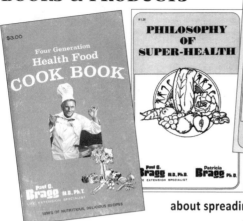

Four Generation Health Food COOK BOOK — $3.00

PHILOSOPHY OF SUPER-HEALTH

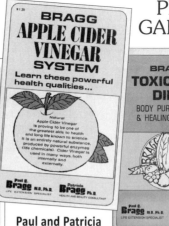

BRAGG APPLE CIDER VINEGAR SYSTEM — Learn these powerful health qualities...

Natural Apple Cider Vinegar is proving to be one of the greatest aids to health and long life known to science. It is an entirely natural substance, produced by powerful enzymes (life chemicals). Cider Vinegar is used in many ways, both internally and externally.

BRAGG TOXICLESS DIET — BODY PURIFICATION & HEALING SYSTEM

Paul and Patricia are passionate about spreading the message of health to the world.

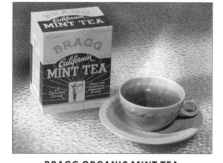

BRAGG TAVA
A delicious chocolate-flavored beverage. Contains vitamins A, B, C, B2, B6 and Iron.

Patricia Bragg carries on her father's Health Legacy that he started over 100 years ago.

Love makes the World go 'round.

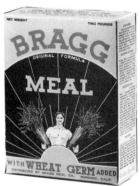

BRAGG MEAL CEREAL
Bragg was first to put wheat germ and 7 grains together for a delicious hot cereal.

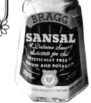

BRAGG SANSAL
A great Salt Substitute. This product was approved by Los Angeles Heart Assoc.

BRAGG 'E' WHEAT GERM OIL
Wheat germ oil with high Vitamin 'E' potency. Includes Omega-3 and Omega-6.

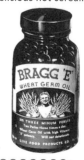

BRAGG ORGANIC MINT TEA
First Organic Herb Teas in America.

"Our lives have completely turned around! Our family is feeling so healthy, we must tell you about it."– Gene & Joan Zollner, parents of 11, Washington

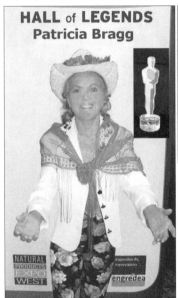

HALL of LEGENDS
Patricia Bragg

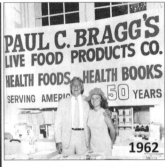

PAUL C. BRAGG'S LIVE FOOD PRODUCTS CO.
HEALTH FOODS – HEALTH BOOKS
SERVING AMERICA 50 YEARS

1962

Paul C. Bragg with Patricia, celebrating over 50 years of Bragg Health Products, Books & Crusading worldwide, spreading Health around the world.

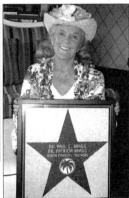

"Palm Spring Walk of Stars" – Patricia with Bragg Star.

Natural Foods Expo in Anaheim with 65,000 attendees from around the world honored Patricia Bragg and her father Paul C. Bragg as treasured Health Food Industry Legends.

BRAGG's 100th Anniversary Celebration

Mrs. Jack LaLanne

Patricia Bragg

2012

100 Year Anniversary Party celebrated at the Natural Foods Expo in Anaheim

Patricia, Staff & 1,000 Friends celebrated our 100 years of Bragg Healthy Products, Books & Health Crusading! We are proud Pioneers in this Big Health Industry that is helping to keep the world healthier! With Blessings of Health, Peace & Love to You!

Patricia

Bragg Hawaii Exercise Class was founded by Worldwide Health Crusader and Fitness Legend, Dr. Paul C. Bragg. He wanted to create a dynamic, Free Community Exercise Class, and he often taught these classes himself for many years. Patricia Bragg continues her father's health legacy by supporting the Bragg Exercise Class and participates in the class whenever she is in Hawaii.

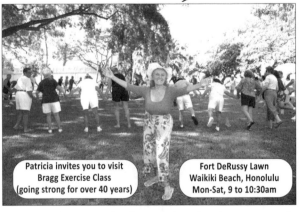

Patricia invites you to visit Bragg Exercise Class (going strong for over 40 years)

Fort DeRussy Lawn Waikiki Beach, Honolulu Mon-Sat, 9 to 10:30am

"Please make a record of your family history & background. Take pictures – make your own 'Photo Gallery'. Take videos – make movies of your children, spouse, mother and father, family gatherings, etc. These memories are precious & important to save for future generations." – Patricia Bragg

Index

Index

D (continued)

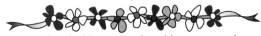

Prayer is the mortar that holds our soul and house together. – Sister Teresa

Index

Roses are God's autograph of beauty, fragrance and love.
– Paul C. Bragg, N.D., Ph.D.

Peace is not a season, it is a way of life.

Index

Through our actions and deeds, rather than promises, let us display the essence of love – perfect harmony in motion! – Philip Glyn, Welsh Poet

The Miracle of Fasting - Proven Throughout History

BY PAUL C. BRAGG, N.D., PH.D.
and PATRICIA BRAGG

In this newly revised best-seller, known to millions as the "bible of fasting" health pioneers and researchers Paul C. Bragg and Patricia Bragg teach why this ancient practice is key to health and energy, and critical to longevity and ageless vitality, due to our toxic environment and the stress of our daily lives. They share a detailed, step-by-step approach, accessible and informative for both beginners and experienced fasters. Our bodies must process not only our food and water, but the air we breathe, and whatever chemicals they may contain. Since detoxification and digestion take more energy than even strenuous athletic pursuits, fasting allows the mind and body to rest, renew and regenerate, to come into harmony and balance, and release the effects of stimulating foods like caffeine and sugars. The goal of fasting, say the authors, is to allow for the mind and body to self-heal. This concise, tightly edited *The Miracle of Fasting* is filled with personal stories of Paul C. Bragg's travels around the world, including a fasting journey in India with Mahatma Gandhi.

Healthy Heart - Learn the Facts

BY PAUL C. BRAGG, N.D., PH.D.
and PATRICIA BRAGG

Heart disease claims more American lives than any other illness and is the number one cause of death for women. World-renowned health pioneers Paul C. Bragg and Patricia Bragg teach time-tested, proven strategies for healing and maintaining a healthy heart for a long, active life! In a world filled with technological wizardry and products, the human heart still outperforms them all. That is – if that human heart is kept healthy. That is what the trailblazers Paul C. Bragg and Patricia Bragg have done in this book, sharing simple suggestions for lifestyle changes, nutritional support and exercises that will keep this most miraculous machine, your body, healthy and strong. You will learn how the heart works and how and why coronary disease is preventable and reversible. The authors provide an easy-to-follow blueprint for heart health that includes stress-release techniques, affirming that a positive mental outlook on life is a major element of heart health. The Braggs are legendary in the field of nutrition and health, and this newly revised and edited edition is a foundation of The Bragg Healthy Lifestyle. It is one of the most comprehensive heart health books on the market today.

194

Building Powerful Nerve Force & Positive Energy - Reduce Stress, Worry and Anger

BY PAUL C. BRAGG, N.D., PH.D.
and PATRICIA BRAGG

What is Nerve Force and why should you care about it? According to mental health trailblazers Paul C. Bragg and Patricia Bragg, "Nerve Force" is a type of life energy stored in the nerves, muscles, organs, and brain. The more Nerve Force you have, the quicker you can re-charge it, and the healthier, happier, and more satisfying a life you will lead. If you suffer from burnout, stress, fatigue, anxiety, insomnia or depression, this book is for you! We know that the ability to feel joy and peace is essential to a complete experience of vitality and wellness. Our thoughts, our attitudes, our outlook, and our emotional well-being are all dependent on having a powerful "Nerve Force." Just like any muscle that we can develop and strengthen, we can build our Nerve Force so that we are resilient, relaxed, and calm, even during times of stress. Paul C. Bragg and Patricia Bragg show you how with simple mental exercises and suggestions for specific foods that replenish your Nerve Force, as well as foods that deplete it, in this newly revised edition of *Building Powerful Nerve Force & Positive Energy* the father-daughter team explains to readers the reward of paying attention to the energy that is responsible for not only our physical capabilities and our vital body functions, but our ability to process information and feel centered and grounded, no matter what life throws at us. They teach us that maintaining a healthy Nerve Force, leads to a balanced and fruitful life.

Super Power Breathing - For Optimum Health & Healing

BY PAUL C. BRAGG, N.D., PH.D.
and PATRICIA BRAGG

Do you sometimes find that you are panting instead of breathing? Many of us do! This can cause headaches, anxiety, fatigue, and brain fog. The quality of our breath determines the quality of our life! This book teaches us how to breathe in a way that replenishes the body with the oxygen it so deeply craves. "The more effectively we breathe, the more effectively we live," write the authors, world-renowned health pioneers Paul C. Bragg and Patricia Bragg. "Super Power Breathing can make your life-force stronger, calmer and smarter." The Super Power Breathing program has been followed by Olympic athletes and millions of Bragg followers, and is filled with simple exercises for energizing and rejuvenating your breath, and your whole body. Research shows that we use only one-fourth to one-half of our lung capacity with each breath. This starves our body much like if we are depriving it of food. We are slowly robbing our body of its most vital, invisible nourishment – oxygen. In its newly revised form, the Bragg Super Power Breathing Program will give you all the tools you need to shift from shallow breathing to taking deep, oxygen-filled, life-giving breaths!

Authored by America's First Family of Health
Live Longer – Healthier – Stronger Self-Improvement Library

Water - The Shocking Truth

BY PAUL C. BRAGG, N.D., PH.D.
and PATRICIA BRAGG

The water you drink can literally make or break your health. The purity of our water is the most critical element in maintaining radical vitality, and healing from illness and disease. In this newly revised edition of *Water: The Shocking Truth*, health crusaders Paul C. Bragg and Patricia Bragg reveal the dangers of tap water, which research shows can be responsible for many ailments, due to the addition of dangerous chemicals such as fluoride and chlorine. In this book, the trailblazing father-daughter team teach the many functions water performs in the body, from regulating the various systems to flushing the body of waste and toxins. But what if the substance we use to cleanse our bodies is itself polluted? With the mandatory fluoridation of water in the municipal water systems, the authors assert that has been the case for decades. Added to the public water supply to prevent tooth decay starting in the 1950s, fluoride has long been known to be a toxin, used in pesticides and rat poisons. Learn what types of water are optimal to drink, how and why to detox your body with nature's most life-giving liquid, and the health-and-life-saving value of installing a water filter in your shower!

Bragg Back & Foot Fitness Program - Keys to a Pain-Free Back & Strong Healthy Feet

BY PAUL C. BRAGG, N.D., PH.D.
and PATRICIA BRAGG

If you are suffering with back or foot pain, look no further for a comprehensive program that will restore health to the parts of your body that carry you through life! Remember when we were children, and we had the kind of energy and flexibility to play for hours? Agile and active, we could twist, bend, stretch and climb with little effort. However, hours looking at a computer screen, a sedentary lifestyle and poor posture can take their toll. Eventually our backs start to hurt and cramp with every movement, and our feet ache after just a short walk. We start feeling "old." In *Bragg Back & Foot Fitness Program*, the father-daughter team of world-renowned health pioneers, Paul C. Bragg and Patricia Bragg teach how to speed the healing of injuries and develop a strong and flexible back and healthy feet, rejuvenating and re-energizing our bodies in the process. The trailblazing health experts who brought wellness and vitality to millions, including fitness guru Jack LaLanne, outline the keys to a healthy spine, pain-free back and bunion-free feet through nutritional support and clearly illustrated, simple exercises, as well as other tips for posture and massage. Paul and Patricia Bragg reveal the healing properties of herbs, effective ways to practice foot reflexology, how to deal with arthritis, athlete's foot, plantar fasciitis, and foot problems caused by diabetes. By following the authors' Back and Foot Care Program, you can begin to treat your body as Mother Nature intended you to, and creating painless feet, a strong back and a powerful body will begin!

PATRICIA BRAGG
Health Crusader and "Angel of Health and Healing"

Author, Lecturer, Nutritionist, Health & Lifestyle Educator to World Leaders, Hollywood Stars, Singers, Athletes & Millions.

Patricia is a life-long health advocate and activist, admired internationally for her passionate work promoting healthy living. For many years she traveled the world, teaching The Bragg Healthy Lifestyle for physical, spiritual, emotional health and joy. She was invited to give lectures, visited radio shows, was profiled in magazines and appealed to people of all ages, nationalities and walks-of-life. Together with Paul, she co-authored a collection of ten books, with inspiration and techniques for living a long, vital, happy life. Now in her 90s and living on an organic farm in California, Patricia herself is a testament to these teachings and the sparkling symbol of health, perpetual youth and radiant energy.

PAUL C. BRAGG, N.D., Ph.D.
Life Extension Specialist • World Health Crusader
Lecturer and Advisor to Olympic Athletes, Royalty, Stars & Millions.
Originator of Health Food Stores & Founder of Health Movement Worldwide

Paul C. Bragg was at the forefront of the modern health movement, having inspired generations to turn toward wellness. At a young age, Paul turned his own health around by developing an eating, breathing and exercise program to build strength and vitality. From this life-changing experience, he pledged to dedicate the rest of his life to promoting a healthy lifestyle. He opened one of the country's first health food stores, which eventually led to the creation of the Bragg Live Foods company. With a devoted following, Paul traveled giving lectures and sharing his expertise, while serving as an advisor to athletes and movie stars alike. Even Jack LaLanne, the original television fitness guru, credited Paul with having introduced him to the importance of healthy living. In addition to the books Paul wrote with Patricia, they co-hosted television and radio shows and worked together to bring wellness to the world. Paul himself excelled in athletics, loved the ocean and the outdoors, and radiated with health and a warm smile.

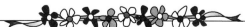

Patricia inspires you to Renew, Rejuvenate and Revitalize your Life with "The Bragg Healthy Lifestyle" Books. Millions have benefitted from these life-changing philosophies with a longer, healthier, happier life!

Take Time for 12 Things

1. Take time to **Work** –
   it is the price of success.

2. Take time to **Think** –
   it is the source of power.

3. Take time to **Play** –
   it is the secret of youth.

4. Take time to **Read** –
   it is the foundation of knowledge.

5. Take time to **Worship** –
   it is the highway of reverence and
   washes the dust of earth from our eyes.

6. Take time to **Help and Enjoy Friends** –
   it is the source of happiness.

7. Take time to **Love and Share** –
   it is the one sacrament of life.

8. Take time to **Dream** –
   it hitches the soul to the stars.

9. Take time to **Laugh** –
   it is the singing that helps life's loads.

10. Take time for **Beauty** –
    it is everywhere in nature.

11. Take time for **Health** –
    it is the true wealth and treasure of life.

12. Take time to **Plan** –
    it is the secret of being able to have time
    for the first 11 things.

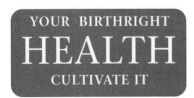
YOUR BIRTHRIGHT
HEALTH
CULTIVATE IT

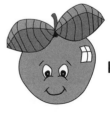

**Have an
Apple
Healthy Life!**

3 John 2

*Teach me thy way, LORD, lead me in a straight path,
because of my oppressors. – Psalm 27:11*